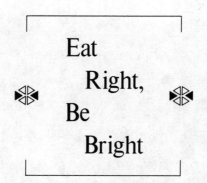

Eat
Right,
Be
Bright

Eat Right, Be Bright

ARTHUR WINTER, M.D.,

and

RUTH WINTER

ST. MARTIN'S PRESS · NEW YORK

**To Samantha Rose, may she always
be bright and eat right**

This book describes current research and theories about the effect of diet on brain function. Before you make any radical changes in your diet, consult your own physician.

Names and other identifying characteristics in this book's case histories have been changed to protect privacy.

Design by Jeremiah B. Lighter

Library of Congress Cataloging-in-Publication Data

Winter, Arthur, 1922-
    Eat right, be bright.

    1. Intellect—Physiological aspects. 2. Nutrition.
3. Brain. I. Winter, Ruth, 1930- . II. Title.
QP398.W56 1988   612'.82   88-1931
ISBN 0-312-01761-8

First Edition
10 9 8 7 6 5 4 3 2 1

Contents

Acknowledgments

THE AUTHORS WISH to thank the following for their willingness to share the results of their research and their expertise: Karl Anderson, M.D., Professor of Preventive Medicine, University of Texas Medical Center, Galveston, TX; Herman Baker, Ph.D., Director, Division of Nutrition and Metabolism, University of Medicine and Dentistry, New Jersey Medical School, Newark, New Jersey; L. Barry Goss, Ph.D., Director Enviromental Sciences Department, Battelle Institute, Columbus, Ohio; Jane Hershey, Executive Director, Feingold Association of the United States; Sarah Leibowitz, Ph.D., Department of Neuropharmacology, Rockefeller University, New York, New York; Thomas Sobotka, Ph.D., Center for Food Safety and Applied Nutrition, U.S. Food and Drug Administration; Hugh Tilson, Ph.D., Director of the Neurobehavorial Section of The National Insitute of Enviromental Health Sciences, Laboratory of Behavior and Neurological Toxicology; Betty Li, Ph.D., U.S. Department of Agriculture Nutrients Analysis Laboratory; Paul Lachance, Ph.D., Professor of Food Science, Rutgers University; Alexander Schauss, Ph.D., Editor-in-Chief, *International Journal of Biosocial Research;* Bernard Weiss, Ph.D., Professor of Toxicology and Deputy Director of The Enviromental Health Sciences Center, University of Rochester School of Medicine; Barbara Anderson, senior editor, St. Martin's Press, who worked diligently to help us translate this often difficult material; and the librarians at St. Barnabas Medical Center, Livingston, New Jersey: Alma Christine Connor, Sylvia Barasso, and Louise Noll.

Introduction

W HEN WE TOURED the country promoting our book, *Build Your Brain Power: The Latest Techniques to Preserve, Restore and Improve Your Brain's Potential,* published by St. Martin's Press in 1986, the one question everyone asked us was, "Which foods are good for the brain?"

The concept that diet can affect the condition of the body is not new. Ever since a Scottish naval surgeon cured scurvy by giving lemons and limes to sailors (forever after known as "limeys"), modern physicians have accepted the fact that *major* nutritional deficiencies can lead to severe alterations in behavior. But the idea that *minor* vitamin and mineral deficiencies can affect the condition of the body or brain, or can alter one's mood or ability to perform, is highly controversial. It is only recently that modern scientists have begun to believe that specific foods may affect our brains and hence our thoughts and behavior. This belief was triggered primarily by the discovery of neurotransmitters, the chemical agents that send messages between brain cells, and the discovery that neurotransmitters are derived from the food we eat.

The subject of food and its effects on the brain is also controversial because the interaction is so complicated and because so much is unknown. Start with the simple questions of why we eat, when we eat, and why we choose the foods we do. Most of us eat three meals a day—breakfast, lunch, and dinner. But what about coffee breaks and snacks after school, in front of the TV, and at bedtime? Are we hungry or do we eat out of habit, boredom, or the need for comfort?

Where are the hunger and satiety centers in the brain and how much voluntary control do we have over our choices of food? Are the eating disorders anorexia (in which there is self-starvation) and obesity (in which there is eating beyond need) culturally or biochemically induced?

There are chemical additives, intentional and unintentional, present in our food and drink. These additives may affect the brain. Certainly, no one would disagree that lead in the diet is toxic to brain cells, but what

about color additives? Artificial sweeteners? Sugars? Antioxidants? More
than ten thousand chemicals in the marketplace have yet to be tested for
their possibly toxic effects on the brain.

Therapeutic uses of food date back at least several thousand years to
ancient Egypt, where onions were recommended to induce sleep, almonds and cabbage to prevent hangovers, lemons to protect against the
evil eye, and salt to stimulate passion.[1] The ancient Greeks also staunchly
believed that diet was an integral part of the treatment of both physical
and psychological illness.[2]

Folk medicine is rich in food prescriptions. Who hasn't heard that
eating oysters will enhance one's sexual desire and performance? This
may be just myth, but in fact oysters are rich in zinc and scientists have
discovered that a zinc deficiency interferes with sexual function.[3]

The brain/food link is not new to modern man, either. We know from
experience that we can use food to alter our moods. Caffeine is the most
common psychoactive (mind- or mood-altering) drug in the world. Ice
cream and candy are typically used as rewards or consolations. Steak and
potatoes make some men feel more manly, just as losing weight helps
raise a woman's self-esteem.

The American Heart Association, the American Cancer Society, and
the federal government made news in the 1980s by recommending a
change in diet to prevent illness. They advised eating more carbohydrates, less fatty meat, and more fish, particularly the deep sea varieties
which contain certain oils that lower cholesterol. Eight hundred years
ago, Maimonides, a famous Jewish physician who practiced in Cor-
dova, Spain, recommended: "Bread is a basic food. Meats should be
very lean and trimmed of all fat. . . . like meat, fish should be lean, the
deep-sea varieties are best. The ideal light-meal to make a person suffering upper respiratory distress is chicken soup."[4] Maimonides and his
contemporaries also believed that humans could modulate their moods
and appetites according to circumstances by using specific food items.
Today it is being rediscovered that diet does indeed affect thought and
behavior.

Although a tremendous amount of research is in progress concerning
the effects of diet on the brain and behavior, the correlations are often
hard to prove because behavioral changes are subtle and it is confounding factors such as culture and stress are difficult to control.

Food represents tradition, reward, love. It is the focal point of most social gatherings. It is a cultural obsession on which Americans spend millions of dollars each year on books, devices, and special diets.

Nevertheless, as anyone who has had a hangover from too much alcohol or irritability due to hunger knows, what we eat and drink can influence how our brains function and, subsequently, our intellect and our behavior.

This book, written by a neurosurgeon and a science writer, describes the burgeoning research on the effects of diet on the brain and, conversely, of the brain on diet. We hope it will give you not only food for thought but also thoughts about your food, because you really are what you eat.

—ARTHUR WINTER, M.D.,
AND RUTH WINTER, B.A.

◁ 1 ▷

The Brain/Food Connection

YOUR BRAIN is a chemical factory that produces dozens of different psychoactive drugs. These self-made compounds affect your intelligence, memory, and mood. The starter materials for these brain chemicals come from the foods you eat.

Your brain is the most important part of your nervous system—the captain of its organization. For your body to survive, your nervous system must be nourished and maintained.

Your brain, by weight alone, comprises 90 percent of your central nervous system. There is also a long extension of your brain descending inside your neck and backbone, known as the spinal cord. From both your brain and your spinal cord, nerves go out to your sensory organs: your eyes, ears, and nose. Your nerves also go out to your muscles, your skin, and all of the other organs of your body.

One of the major functions of your central nervous system is communication—communication within its various parts and with the outside world. Your brain has its own private "postal system." Each individual nerve cell, or neuron, can communicate with thousands of other cells by chemical messengers called *neurotransmitters.* Your body creates these brainy postal "employees" from substances in your diet. They deliver their information between neurons in the brain and elsewhere in the body electrically by "wire" or chemically, like a bottle tossed in the ocean. Within the neurons, signals are sent predominantly by wire (electrically); conversely, the signals that are transmitted from one neuron to another "shoot the rapids" to carry their messages across the gaps between neurons—a process called *synapsis.* Since neurons do not touch one another, nature provided a chemical "letter-carrying" system as well as an electronic mail setup.

1

Your brain's postal service has an amazing capacity to deliver. It was once believed that messages could be sent only between adjoining nerves. Now it is known that nerves can issue substances that travel throughout the body, affecting other nerves at distant sites. It has also been recently discovered that a single nerve is capable of sending out several messages, not just one, as previously believed.

You can alter the levels and functions of these neurotransmitters with drugs such as antidepressants, which elevate your mood, tranquilizers,

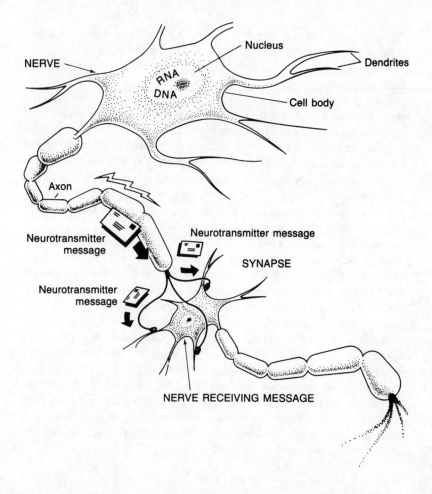

which calm you down, and stimulants, which increase your alertness. Your diet can also alter your mood and your ability to think—perhaps not as dramatically as drugs but usually a lot more safely.

The line between foods and drugs in prevention and/or cure of human maladies is fading. You consume foods, which are composed of a variety of chemicals, in relatively large amounts to supply your body with energy, regulate its processes, and repair its tissues. You take drugs, which are chemicals, in small quantities for a specific purpose, such as to kill pain or to soothe anxiety. Thanks to new research capabilities, it is becoming increasingly clear that there is something to the old idea that "food is your best medicine."

Today there are three major areas in which the disciplines of nutrition and pharmacology interact and are of vital importance to your brain's functioning: (1) vitamins and minerals, in the prevention or treatment of conditions or diseases; (2) drug-nutrient interactions, in which food can enhance or retard the effects of drugs and vice versa; and (3) foods that act as drugs on the brain. The raw materials for those self-produced brain "drugs" are proteins in the diet. Modern neuroscientists are proving in the laboratory what the ancients only surmised—that certain foods do affect the brain.

Take bananas, for example. In ancient India, bananas were called "the fruit of wise men." There is even a legend that claims it was the banana, not the apple, that was the forbidden fruit in the Garden of Eden. In any case, it was one of the first fruits cultivated by humans.[2] The banana's botanical name, *Musa sapientum* (roughly translated as "smart herb"), is attributed to the Greek philosopher Pliny, who noted, "sages reposed beneath its shade and ate of its fruit."

What did the wise men of the past know that modern scientists are only now confirming in their laboratories about the effect of this particular food on the human brain? An average small banana contains about 81 calories, 1 gram of protein, 21.1 grams of carbohydrate, 8 milligrams of calcium, 25 milligrams of phosphorous, 352 milligrams of potassium, and 1 milligram of sodium. It is 99.8 percent fat-free and has 180 international units of vitamin A, 10 milligrams of vitamin C, and two neurotransmitter materials: 15 micrograms per gram weight of serotonin and 1.62 milligrams of tryptophan.

Later in this book we will discuss in more detail many of the components in a banana, but just briefly they provide the following benefits:

- **Carbohydrates** (sugars and starches), the material from which glucose, the major fuel for your brain, is derived. Ingesting carbohydrates can also affect your mood and cravings.

- **Potassium,** vital to the transmission of messages between your nerves.

- **Low sodium,** a benefit for those with sodium-caused water retention due to high blood pressure or kidney problems. Water retention can produce symptoms ranging from irritability to coma.

- **Vitamin A,** which is necessary for keen eyesight. Through eyesight, of course, we gain most of the information we feed our brains. A deficiency of vitamin A has also been found, at least in laboratory animals, to affect balance and cause abnormalities in taste and smell, two senses intimately involved in eating.[3]

- **Vitamin C,** which has been linked to the production of *dopamine,*[4] another neurotransmitter in your brain and one that is necessary for coordinated movements, and to the production of *tyrosine,* another neurotransmitter. Tyrosine serves as a building block for *epinephrine* and *norepinephrine,* neurotransmitters involved in strong emotions and alertness (see chart on page 9). Vitamin C also participates in the processing of glucose, the brain's primary food.[5]

- **Phosphorous,** essential in all energy-producing reactions of cells, including brain cells.

- **Serotonin,** a neurotransmitter that inhibits secretions in the digestive tract and stimulates smooth muscles. It is an important regulator of both mood and appetite. Low levels of serotonin have been linked to depression.[6]

- **Tryptophan,** a raw material for brain chemicals involved in mood and sleep.

It may be smart to include bananas in your diet, but bananas alone will not make you smart. Even though many of the observations made by ancient sages and ordinary people about the impact of certain foods on brain function may prove to be well-founded, the research today concerning diet and the brain is often complicated by other factors, such as culture, heredity, and personal experience. The results of experiments to correlate diet and brain function, therefore, are often inconclusive and controversial.

What is agreed on is that in order for a chemical messenger in your brain to be manufactured from a substance in food, four things must happen:

1. The substance must be absorbed through your gastrointestinal tract.

2. It must be carried by your blood to a specific area in your brain.

3. It must be converted by enzymes, the workhorses of your body, into a specific neurotransmitter.

4. Once manufactured, the neurotransmitter must be stored in the proper place and be available for release when needed.

At first, scientists did not believe that foods could alter the levels of neurotransmitters, because the manufacture of these highly potent brain chemicals must be exquisitely regulated; any interference with them can cause all sorts of problems, ranging from memory loss and depression to muscle paralysis and inability to speak. It is now known, however, that foods can modify the production of neurotransmitters and result in changes in brain function, mood, and behavior that are often predictable.

You do not have to be a neuroscientist to make a cause-and-effect assumption about something you ate and its influence on your thinking and behavior. A good example is a person who suffers from panic attacks. The condition, which is believed to have a combined physical and emotional cause, produces a feeling of impending doom where there is no real danger. Medical specialists who treat such patients report that invariably, on their own, the patients had stopped drinking beverages containing caffeine because they recognized the association between their ingestion of caffeine and their symptoms. As discussed in chapter 8, caffeine can trigger panic attacks.[7]

Alcohol consumption offers another obvious example of the effects of ingested substances on brain function. Have you ever been drunk or even slightly tipsy? What do you think happened to your ability to think clearly? The alcohol you ingested affected or damaged your brain cells.

When ingested by a pregnant woman, alcohol can cripple the brain of her unborn child. But most of the time, the effects of food and drink on brain function are subtle and occur over a long period of time.

Your brain consumes a whopping 50 percent of your body's fuel, glucose, which is obtained from food. Since your brain is the most important part of your nervous system, all of your other organs will undergo sacrifice to keep your brain going when you are under severe stress or when you are eating an energy-deficient, nutritionally poor diet.

More than sixty neurotransmitters have been identified at this writing, and it is believed that many more have yet to be discovered. Neurotransmitters are manufactured from the raw materials in food by the nerve cell body. They then travel down the *axon*—the long part of the nerve that looks like a telephone pole—and are stored in tiny capsules at the end of the axon to await a signal to spurt information (synapse) to another nerve cell across the gap.

Neurotransmitter messages are received at sites called *receptors,* which are specicifically made for them. A particular neurotransmitter fits into a certain receptor like a piece in a jigsaw puzzle.

A neurotransmitter may cause a recipient nerve cell to fire a message, or it may discourage it from doing so and then disappear in a matter of milliseconds. In contrast, the neurotransmitter may order a long-lasting

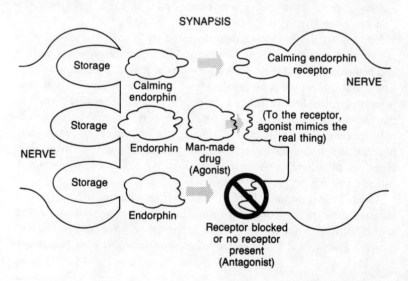

change in the receiving cell, perhaps switching on genes that create the production of a new transmitter or receptor.

Recently it has been discovered that a single nerve cell may release two or more neurotransmitters or may switch from producing one neurotransmitter to producing another. Thus, a single nerve cell can send different messages at different times, depending on what is going on in the body and what food, drink, and drugs have been ingested. The impact goes well beyond the single nerve cell and can affect the entire body. Consider the neurotransmitter called *endorphin*, for example. The most familiar of the self-made brain "drugs," its name derives from the Greek *endon-* and *morphine*, meaning "morphine from within." Endorphins can sedate, cause euphoria, or kill pain, depending on where they are sent and where they are received.

Foreign chemicals—those that are not manufactured in the body and that affect the brain, such as drugs and certain nutrients—can act in two ways. They may mimic the natural neurotransmitter and trigger a response by the nerve cell, or they may take up space on the receptor but fail to elicit a response in the cell. In so doing, they also prevent natural neurotransmitters from binding to the receptor. In the first case, drugs that mimic the real thing and turn on the cell are called *agonists*. In the second case, they are called *antagonists* or *blockers*. In fact, all drugs used to treat mental illness function by either mimicking or blocking the action of natural transmitters. Long-term use of psychoactive substances mimics the manufacture of a natural neurotransmitter; thus, the production of the natural chemical may shut down. When the mimicry is stopped, there may be an insufficient amount of the natural neurotransmitter, and severe withdrawal symptoms may occur, such as the d.t.'s (delirium tremens) of alcoholics or the multiple mental and physical symptoms of the heroin addict.

The same process is at work in people who suddenly stop drinking large quantities of products containing caffeine, such as coffee or colas. Their receptor sites for the caffeine molecules are empty, waiting for a jolt that never comes. As a result, they suffer headaches, malaise, and other symptoms.

The blocking or destruction of certain receptor sites is thought to play a major role in the mind-destroying Alzheimer's disease and even in the common memory problems of healthy people as they grow older. The neurons that produce and receive the neurotransmitter *acetylcholine*, which is vital to memory, are affected. It is believed that the loss or malfunctioning of these receptors may account for much of forgetfulness, in the same way that women who had "Twilight Sleep" while giving birth literally forgot the pain because the memory receptors in their brains were blocked by the drug scopolamine. Researchers are studying *acetylcholinesterase,* the enzyme that destroys acetylcholine, in hope of stopping the destruction of this neurotransmitter and its receptors.[8] One of the avenues of research is the study of *choline,* a substance found in concentrated amounts in egg yolks and present in meat and some cereals. Choline serves as a raw material for acetylcholine.

Blocking or destroying a neurotransmitter is one problem, but once a neurotransmitter binds to a receptor, it must eventually be deactivated so that information transmission can resume. If not, we would have uncoordinated movements or paralysis. A general "turn off" for neurotransmission is believed to be a neurotransmitter called *gammaaminobutyric acid* (GABA). When GABA is released from a nerve cell and binds to the receptor of another, the recipient nerve cell is inhibited from firing its own message. A muscle relaxant such as Valium is thought to work by making GABA turn off nerves involved in spewing out anxiety messages. GABA is found in high concentrations in the brain but, oddly, seems to be absent from the rest of the body.[9] A number of food ingredients, as described later in this book, are believed to affect the amount of GABA in the brain.

Some neurotransmitters are not turned off by GABA but are deactivated by their own nerve cells, which suck them back in. Drugs such as cocaine and amphetamines act by interfering with this re-uptake mechanism. Other neurotransmitters are inactivated by special workhorse enzymes. The neurotransmitters dopamine, epinephrine, and norepinephrine, which are involved in movement, blood pressure, and mood, are destroyed by the enzyme *monoamine oxidase* (MAO). People taking MAO-inhibitors (drugs for treating depression) are warned against eating foods like herring or drinking wine because these substances are high in *tyramine,* the raw material for epinephrine (see pages 119–121). The combination of high levels of epinephrine made by the body from the tyramine in ingested foods and the lack of epinephrine's turn-off enzyme, MAO, can send a person's blood pressure skyrocketing and cause a stroke.

Research into neurotransmitters and their receptors is in its infancy,

NEUROTRANSMITTER MAIN MENU

NEUROTRANSMITTER	FUNCTION (Proven or believed)
Acetylcholine	Aids memory, transmits signals
Epinephrine (adrenaline)	Stimulates, prepares body for stress
Norepinephrine (noradrenaline)	Stimulates, promotes appetite
Amino acids	
GABA	Turns off nerve signals
Glutamic acid	Catalyst
Glycine	Inhibits signals
Dopamine	Initiates movement
Substance P	Alerts to pain
Serotonin	Calms, affects appetite
Hypothalamic-releasing hormones	
Thyrotropin-releasing hormone (TRH)	Affects energy and mood
Luteinizing hormone-releasing hormone (LHRH)	Stimulates sexual appetite
Somatostatin (SRIF)	Affects growth and energy
Enkephalins and endorphins	Pain killers
Neuropeptide Y	Affects eating behavior
Vasoactive intestinal peptide (VIP)	Affects thirst, blood pressure
Cholecystokinin (CCK)	Affects appetite
Adrenocorticotropic hormone (ACTH)	Affects energy
Pituitary hormones	
Insulin	Metabolism of carbohydrates
Vasopressin	Affects thirst, blood pressure

TABLE—*Continued*

NEUROTRANSMITTER	FUNCTION (Proven or Believed)
Oxytocin	Affects hunger, glucose
Angiotensin	Affects blood pressure
Glucagon	Affects hunger, glucose
Corticotropin-releasing factor (CRF)	Affects appetite, stress
Growth-hormone-releasing hormone (GHRH)	Affects sexual appetite
Calcium messenger system	Triggers changes in sending and receiving between nerve cells
Nerve growth factor (NGF)	Promotes maintenance and repair in nervous system
Substance YY	Carbohydrate craving

but the knowledge that there are receptors in the brain and throughout the body that recognize and bind specific neurotransmitters, hormones, and drugs is the foundation of much of the current search for new medications as well as efforts to increase the understanding of how food ingredients affect the brain. Neurotransmitter-receptor interaction directly influences your mood, appetite, blood pressure, pain perception, coordination, and every other function of your brain. Conversely, what you eat and drink affects the production and function of your brain's neurotransmitters. There is an exquisite balance in your brain's nervous system—a network of chemical keys and locks and switches that turns things on and off. These chemicals are both made from and influenced by diet. A neuron is like any other cell in your body in that it needs to receive oxygen and food and eliminate waste products. In the next chapter, we will describe some of the research now in progress involving amino acids, the very building blocks of the neurotransmitters that come from food, and how these bits of protein may affect your brain and your behavior.

Amino Acids: Messengers of the Mind

How much would you pay for a magic potion of twenty chemicals that would build your brain power by enhancing your ability to think and remember, by allowing you to sleep and wake easily, and by aiding your coordination? You could pay as much as thirty dollars or more for a bottle of amino acids, as some stores are now charging, or you could obtain the same chemicals by paying five dollars for a bowl of chili or for pizza with cheese or even thirty dollars for a steak dinner.

Actually, amino acids are as priceless as they are powerful. They are the body's building blocks from which proteins are constructed. Protein not only creates body tissue—muscles, bones, hair, and nails—it also transports oxygen and carries the genetic code of life to all of your cells. As if that weren't enough, protein is used by your body to manufacture antibodies (disease fighters), hormones (gland messengers), and neurotransmitters (nerve cell messengers). Of the twenty amino acids that go into building the millions of proteins in your body, nine cannot be manufactured by your body in sufficient quantities to sustain growth and health and must be obtained from your diet. These nine are called *essential* amino acids because they are essential for maintaining good health. They are:

Isoleucine	Threonine
Leucine	Tryptophan
Lysine	Valine
Methionine	Histidine (thought to be essential
Phenylalanine	only in children)

11

Other, "nonessential" amino acids can be obtained from your diet or manufactured in your intestines and liver. They are:

Alanine	Glutamic acid
Arginine	Glutamine
Asparagine	Serine
Aspartic acid	Tyrosine
Cystine	Taurine
Glycine	

Your brain is almost completely regulated by amino acids, and their journey from your plate to your head depends on the content of your meals, your physical condition, your activity, and your environment.

When you eat a meal of meat, beans, or any other protein-containing food, digestive enzymes in your stomach and small intestines break apart the protein molecule into "free" amino acids and into small bunches of amino acids, called *peptides,* strung together head-to-tail. Your liver then controls the distribution of amino acids in your blood. As the amino acids move through your bloodstream, your body selects the particular amino acid building blocks it needs for its organs and its functions. That steak you ate, therefore, may become part of your nails or the muscle of your big toe, or it may go to your brain to help get this information you are reading right now across your brain cells.

Your brain uses amino acids to produce enzymes, the "workers" that convert raw materials into useful products. The enzymes, in turn, use amino acids to manufacture neurotransmitters, such as dopamine to help you move and serotonin to calm you down. Each of your brain's neurotransmitters has its own personal enzyme.

Think of a neurotransmitter in your brain as a sentence. The amino acids are the "words" that are strung together in a certain order to form the "sentence." Each sentence, or neurotransmitter, carries a particular message between nerve cells in your brain.

The neurotransmitter sentences are constructed in two ways: (1) Directly from the amino acids in the protein you eat, and (2) indirectly, by causing insulin to be released from your pancreas, which then draws amino acids from your blood and tissues.

There are natural, daily fluctuations in amino acid levels in your blood,[1] but the content of your meals can cause major changes in blood and brain levels of these powerful substances and thus affect your thinking, mood, and behavior.

Amino acids are extremely powerful in small doses and are versatile in changing roles, depending on where they are used in the body. It is not surprising, therefore, that one of the hottest areas in pharmaceutical research today involves amino acids.

That they are essential to your brain and body and are derived from foods, however, does not mean amino acids are harmless and should be taken lightly. The amino acid levels in your body are exquisitely balanced. By overloading your system with one, you can affect the levels of others, which may produce serious adverse effects on your body and brain. For example, in the *American Journal of Psychiatry* reported the case of a man who took up to 4 grams of L-glutamine, a form of the amino acid glutaric acid, every day for three weeks and wound up having grandiose delusions, total insomnia, and an uncontrollable sex drive.[2] These symptoms may appeal to some, but his psychiatrist reported that the patient was also psychotic and had hallucinations. Within a week after the patient was off the supplement, the symptoms cleared. Another man who took L-glutamine, which is easily accessible in health food stores, found himself losing sleep and experiencing hyperactivity and sharper mental activity.[3] In general, he felt very uncomfortable. When he stopped taking the amino acid, his symptoms subsided. Long-term effects of taking L-glutamine as a supplement are of course unknown.

The U.S. Food and Drug Administration (FDA) believes that the ingestion of large amounts of individual amino acids can be harmful and in 1974 it removed amino acids from the agency's Generally Recognized As Safe (GRAS) list. However, the FDA has approved the addition of amino acids to foods for two purposes: fortifying protein-containing foods to improve food value, and treating metabolic disorders related to certain diseases. In the latter case, the FDA considers them "medical foods" These products have to be tested for safety and efficacy as if they were drugs.[4]

Although much remains to be learned about amino acids, the following tables indicate some of their known functions and sources.

A tremendous amount of research is now in progress to determine how amino acids affect brain function and behavior. Literally thousands of scientific papers are presented each year on the subject. The following

ESSENTIAL AMINO ACIDS			
AMINO ACID	FUNCTION IN BODY	COMMERCIAL USES	SOURCES IN DIET
Histidine*	growth nerve function blood vessel dilation	dietary supplement	ham veal shredded wheat beef, round chicken egg noodles cheddar cheese dried milk (nonfat)
Isoleucine	growth	dietary supplement	milk halibut processed cheese chicken macaroni beef, round veal salmon
Leucine	liver function overdose can cause imbalance in other amino acids and may deplete immunity[a]	dietary supplement used in the diagnosis of alcoholism and liver damage	turkey corn grits beef, chuck cottage cheese liver processed cheese milk ham
Lysine	glucose metabolism liver function antibody formation	dietary supplement	milk turkey legumes salmon beef, chuck haddock
Methionine	antidepressant when combined with vitamin B_{12} cell structure and function	"fresh" potato flavoring for chips, soups snacks, salad dressings	milk liver corn grits bread stuffing whole wheat

TABLE—*Continued*

AMINO ACID	FUNCTION IN BODY	COMMERCIAL USES	SOURCES IN DIET
Phenylalanine	with tyrosine, acts as a building block of the neurotransmitter norepinephrine	treatment of multiple sclerosis, spasm, and depression the sweetener aspartame is made with it	whole eggs chicken liver milk cottage and processed cheese chocolate beef pumpernickel bread potato brown rice soy flour noodles
Threonine	prevents buildup of fats in liver (last essential amino acid to be discovered; in 1935)		whole eggs gelatin skim milk turkey hamburger halibut
Tryptophan	building block of neurotransmitter serotonin	treatment of pain, depression, insomnia and appetite control	peanuts oatmeal banana beef, round lamb bouillon swiss cheese almonds milk calf's liver roast turkey Parmesan cheese egg yolk peanut butter egg noodles string beans

| | | | TABLE—*Continued* |
AMINO ACID	FUNCTION IN BODY	COMMERCIAL USES	SOURCES IN DIET
Valine	growth and nitrogen balance	dietary supplement	veal liver dried milk (nonfat) processed cheese beef, round lamb, leg chicken oats corn cereal

*Essential only in children.
[a]See W. R. Beisel, "Malnutrition and the Immune Response," in *Biochemistry of Nutrition*, vol. 1, ed. A. Neuberger and T. H. Jukes (Baltimore: University Park Press, 1979), 1–19.

NONESSENTIAL AMINO ACIDS

AMINO ACID	FUNCTION IN BODY	COMMERCIAL USES	SOURCES IN DIET
Alanine	released by muscles to aid glucose production during fasting	dietary supplement	
Arginine	urine production can produce nausea growth hormone production aid stimulates white blood cell production	"overnight" diet pills being tested as an immunity booster[a]	veal peanuts poultry peanut butter walnuts milk
Asparagine	helps produce urine	diuretic	asparagus peas

AMINO ACID	FUNCTION IN BODY	COMMERCIAL USES	SOURCES IN DIET
Aspartic acid	nitrogen and energy metabolism major neurotransmitter substance	sweetener asparatame is derived from it	sugar beets sugar cane molasses beef
Cystine	promotes wound healing glucose metabolism	treatment for hair loss and brittle nails	beef, chuck and round leg of lamb oatmeal chicken flour milk turkey salmon egg noodles
Glutamic acid	urine production nitrogen and energy metabolism major stimulating neurotransmitter substance	MSG is made from it magnesium salts are used as tranquilizer	Oriental foods containing seaweed foods with MSG or aspartame
Glutamine	aids urine production may aid elasticity in cells	feed additive	wheat flour sugar beets
Glycine	retards fat rancidity	chicken feed additive dietary supplement antacid	gelatin sugar cane

TABLE—*Continued*

AMINO ACID	FUNCTION IN BODY	COMMERCIAL USES	SOURCES IN DIET
Serine	helps produce the neurotrans- mitter acetylcholine	dietary supplement	beef gelatin
Tyrosine	helps produce the neurotrans- mitters norepinephrine, epinephrine, and dopamine helps produce thyroid hormone, which controls metabolism, and melanin, which affects skin and hair color	antistress, blood pressure, and antidepressant medications	peanuts oatmeal cheese chicken beef, round leg of lamb calf's liver bouillon bananas roast turkey milk ham egg noodles egg yolk almonds
Taurine	aids digestion scavenges free radicals nerve stimulation may be essential for fetal and infant brain and nervous system development	biochemical research emulsifying agent	oysters beef mussels liver human milk

[a]See "Beefy Boost for Ailing Immune System," *Medical World News,* 16 February 1981, 34.

section describes some of the more recent findings concerning amino acids and the brain.

Arginine, which plays an important part in the production of urine and is necessary for healing wounds, is the main component of some products touted as "overnight" diet pills. Arginine affects the secretion of growth hormone, which, in turn, supposedly affects appetite—the rationale for its use in appetite-suppressant pills. In large doses it causes nausea, which may be another explanation for its appetite-suppressing quality. The FDA says that arginine is used in clinical settings to measure a patient's secretion of growth hormone, but the amount used is large and it is injected rather than taken orally. Because of its ability to stimulate growth hormone, clinical studies are now underway to see if arginine bolsters immunity in the injured, in patients recovering from operations, and in victims of infections or malignancies. In animal studies, it does stimulate the action of disease-fighting white blood cells.[5]

Methionine, an essential amino acid, has been found to have antidepressant effects when metabolized with vitamin B_{12} into a compound called S-adenosyl methionine (SAM). In several studies this compound was found to be as effective as some antidepressant drugs now widely used, ameliorating symptoms such as guilt, suicidal ideation, slowness of movement, work problems, and lack of interest. It was also reported to be more rapid in taking effect than conventional antidepressant drugs, with many patients showing improvement after four to seven days as compared to the ten days to two weeks it usually takes with other medications. Methionine also seems to be free of side effects. As of this writing it is being clinically tested in the United Kingdom, Italy, and the United States.[6]

The essential amino acid *phenylalanine* is, along with another amino acid, tyrosine, a building block of the brain messenger norepinephrine, which has to do with memory function as well as with sex drive.

An inborn metabolic defect in which there is an inability to process the phenylalanine in food (phenylketonuria, or PKU) leads to mental deterioration and eventually death if phenylalanine is not restricted in the diet. A deficiency of or an inability to utilize phenylalanine has also been linked to the destruction of nerve coverings, which then interferes with their transmission of messages, producing incoordination and other problems, like those seen in multiple sclerosis. A partner in the destruction of the nerve coverings, according to some theories, is an inability to utilize vitamin B_{12}. Therefore, phenylalanine and B_{12} given together show promise in the treatment of multiple sclerosis and related diseases. In a four-year study of patients with multiple sclerosis, D-phenylalanine was given with B_{12}. In varying degrees, the patients experienced a reversal in bladder spasms and the return of muscle control.[7]

Phenylalanine has also been used for weight loss, as an antidepressant, and as an antispasmodic. And the food industry is now injecting eight million pounds of phenylalanine into the food supply each year in the form of the sweetener aspartame.

The nonessential amino acid *serine* is metabolized into choline, which is used to make acetylcholine, the very important neurotransmitter that sparks the sending of messages between cells (see page 8) and that is vital to the ability to remember.

Tyrosine, widely distributed in animal protein, is not considered an essential amino acid because it can be manufactured by the body from phenylalanine. When the enzyme that transforms phenylalanine into tyrosine is not active, the serious inherited disease PKU occurs. As mentioned earlier, PKU causes mental deficiency.

Tyrosine, in turn, is a building block for the nerve messengers epinephrine, norepinephrine, and dopamine, as well as for thyroid hormone and melanin, the dark brown and black skin and hair pigment. Norepinephrine and epinephrine are involved in strong emotions and alertness. Dopamine is involved in movement and mood. Thyroid hormone is necessary for normal metabolism of food and also strongly influence brain function and behavior. Mental retardation occurs in children and mental abnormalities in adults who have insufficient thyroid hormone.

Dr. Alan J. Gelenberg, a psychiatrist at Harvard Medical School, reported that some depressed patients who took tablets of tyrosine, in addition to their regular diet, improved.[8] The tyrosine provided solely by a high-protein diet, however, did not have the same effect.

In another study, this one done at the Massachusetts Institute of Technology (MIT), E. Melamed and his colleagues measured the amino acid levels in eleven healthy young men who consumed a diet containing 113 milligrams of protein per day and who took 100 milligrams per kilogram of body weight per day of L-tyrosine in three equal doses before meals.[9] The men's blood levels of tyrosine rose from .13 to .21 on the day they received the tyrosine. This led to the conclusion that ingesting supplemental tyrosine may increase the tyrosine levels in the brain, thus enabling the brain to manufacture its own neurotransmitters to combat conditions such as parkinsonism, depression, and high blood pressure, in which neurotransmitter deficiencies play a part.

Of all the amino acids, *tryptophan* has perhaps most captured the interest of scientists and lay persons. A tremendous amount of scientific research is in progress with this amino acid, which is a building block for the calming neurotransmitter serotonin. Tryptophan was first isolated in milk in 1901. It is believed to work in partnership with tyrosine (see page 20) in producing not only serotonin but also the stimulating brain messengers dopamine and norepinephrine. Tryptophan is the least abundant essential amino acid present in the average diet.[10]

Laboratory and clinical findings suggest that tryptophan malnutrition and, consequently, tryptophan administration may have important roles in treating some brain and behavior problems.[11] A number of studies have been done on the use of tryptophan and its chemical relatives to treat depression and insomnia. Dr. Ernest Hartmann of the Tufts University School of Medicine, for example, has studied the effects of extra doses of tryptophan on groups of mild insomniacs and normal sleepers.[12] Those who took tryptophan tablets fell asleep more quickly.

Dr. Michael Yogman of the Children's Hospital Medical Center in Boston also showed the sleep-inducing effects of tryptophan. He reported that babies fell asleep faster when a solution of sugar and tryptophan was added to their bottles, but warned against mothers doing their own experimenting with tryptophan.[13] As we have pointed out, amino acids are not innocuous.

In 1971, Richard Wurtman, M.D., an endocrinologist at MIT, and a colleague showed that the levels of tryptophan in the brain directly control how much serotonin the brain will manufacture. Some types of depression are thought to be linked to abnormal serotonin levels. Thus, researchers have postulated that depression might be treated with increased levels of tryptophan, to help the body produce more serotonin. Some studies report benefits, others do not. The tryptophan is given as a pharmaceutical in doses of 2 to 12 grams daily. Even an amount as small as about 25 milligrams can significantly raise serotonin levels in the brain.[14]

Tryptophan has shown some promise as an alternative to stimulant drugs in children with learning disorders, according to researchers at the Ohio State University School of Medicine.[15] Elaine D. Nemzer, M.D., and her colleagues tried one-week courses of tryptophan, tyrosine, amphetamine, and a placebo in fourteen children with attention problems. Amphetamine proved effective. Tryptophan showed promise. The placebo and tyrosine had no effect.

The Ohio State investigators reported that the children's parents said tryptophan worked very well in the home setting. Five of the parents even rated the amino acid higher than amphetamine. The teachers, however, did not see any significant difference in behavior with tryptophan. The researchers theorized that the difference in observations between parents and teachers may be that tryptophan can have a sedating effect that would be more noticeable at home than in school.

While indicating that additional studies would be needed to determine various dosages and long-term effects, the Ohio researchers suggested three possible uses of tryptophan:

1. Where parents have trouble at home with children but schools do not.

2. During summer vacations, when a holiday from stimulation might be desirable.

3. As an evening supplement, when the morning stimulant dose wears off.

There is also a great deal of work in progress concerning tryptophan as an antipain medication. University of Pennsylvania researchers, for example, are testing L-tryptophan to reduce chronic pain in patients recovering from the "nerve virus" shingles or from an accident and have found it "promising."[16]

Dr. Samuel Seltzer and his colleagues at nearby Temple University Health Science Center in Philadelphia are experimenting with tryptophan supplements to increase levels of serotonin in the brain as a means of dulling pain.[17] A four-week, double-blind study was conducted with thirty patients suffering chronic jaw pain radiating down one or more nerves. Half of the patients were given tryptophan, half were not. In a report in the *Journal of Psychiatric Research,* these researchers said that not only was there a reduction in pain among the tryptophan group, there was also a greater tolerance to experimental pain when applied to a tooth. Tryptophan, they concluded, reduced pain sensitivity.

Sold over the counter tryptophan is taken for its calming, sleep-inducing, and pain-relieving effects, presumably due to the production of serotonin. However, tryptophan is neither approved by the FDA nor recognized by the American Medical Association (AMA) as a drug. Megadoses of single amino acids, as pointed out before, can be dangerous. Tryptophan has produced fatty changes in the livers of rats. Because liver metabolism of tryptophan is similar in rats and humans, such findings raise serious questions about long-term supplementation to achieve positive effects as a drug.[18]

In liver cirrhosis (scarring due to disease or alcoholism), for example, there may be a buildup in the brain of tryptophan and, consequently, of serotonin. The brain then goes into the deep sleep known as *coma.* This scenario receives some support from clinical studies in which patients with liver coma were roused by administering amino acids that would counteract tryptophan by competing with it for entry into the brain.

This competition between amino acids to enter the brain explains why certain amino acids may enter the brain when a high-carbohydrate meal rather than a high-protein meal is eaten, even though amino acids are derived from protein. It has to do with the natural defense system called the *blood-brain barrier,* a collection of brain cells that act like secret service agents to protect a "head of state" against assassins and hecklers. Constantly on guard, the blood-brain barrier allows only a certain amount of particular types of amino acids to pass through at one time.[19]

There is competition within each type of amino acid to get past the barrier and into the brain tissue. Once there is "no more room," because its competitors got there first, the blood brain barrier prevents other amino acids from entering. For example, high-protein meals fail to increase the level of tryptophan in the brain because the other amino acids are much more abundant in dietary proteins. The competition for access to the brain, then, becomes weighted against tryptophan.[20] Thus, whether an amino acid in your diet will get to your brain depends not only on the concentration of the amino acid in your diet and blood but also on the concentrations of its amino acid competitors.

Recognition of this phenomenon has already shown promise in therapy with Parkinson's disease patients. More than one and a half million Americans suffer from this devastating nervous disorder, which is characterized by involuntary trembling of the limbs and facial muscles, extreme slowness of movement, and muscular rigidity that makes even simple activities like walking or picking up a book difficult. Levodopa, a drug that raises the level of dopamine in the brain, is a treatment that has freed many Parkinson's patients from the prison of the disease, but it often produces side effects that are as bad as the disease—rapid and unpredictable shifts in movement, ranging from excessive involuntary movements to almost no movements at all.

A number of Parkinson's patients have noted that hot, spicy meals result in violent movements, while meat products or other foods rich in protein make them stiffer and slower. These patients determined that a bland or vegetarian diet causes fewer or less severe symptoms.

The effects of protein on the absorption of levodopa was then studied, and it was discovered that some amino acids may block the absorption of levodopa from the gut or block its entry into the brain.[21] On the other hand, many patients are unable to tolerate levodopa on an empty stomach and experience nausea and vomiting. Thus, patients must often compromise between getting levodopa's full effect by taking it on an empty stomach, and preventing nausea and vomiting by taking it with food.

A Yale Medical School physician, Jonathan H. Pincus, and his associates gave eleven Parkinson's patients a special diet regimen.[22] They were to eat carbohydrates all day and eat proteins only at night. From the time they woke up until 5:00 P.M., the patients ate no meat, poultry, dairy products, legumes, nuts, or baked goods (which contain milk and eggs). After a short time, nine of the patients "experienced a marked relief of Parkinsonian symptoms" as well as a lessening of the side effects often brought on by levodopa.[23] Moreover, eight of these patients were able to reduce their dosage of the medication by an average of 41 percent. Physicians in private practice who read about the results began trying the new therapy on their own patients and are reporting similar success.[24] But when the high-protein meal is eaten in the evening to make up for the lack of protein all day, "patients experience an exacerbation of Parkinsonian symptoms that can last up to three or four hours," Dr. Pincus and his colleagues pointed out. "Nonetheless, the simple measure of avoiding protein during the daytime is allowing patients who suffer from the side effects of levodopa to enjoy hours of near-normal functioning and independence."[25]

So what should you eat to make sure your brain gets the amino acid building blocks it needs to manufacture neurotransmitters in your brain? Your first priority is a diet sufficient in protein. (The word *protein* itself means "of first importance.") Customary intake by Westerners is 100 grams of dietary protein. You contribute about 70 grams of self-made protein per day and you lose about 10 grams per day by elimination of waste. That means you have to process 160 grams of protein per day.

High-quality proteins contain the essential amino acids in an available form and in near-optimal proportions. Animal proteins—sometimes called "complete" proteins—such as eggs, meat, fish, poultry, and dairy products are high-quality proteins. Most plant proteins are deficient in one or more of the essential amino acids, and these amino acids may not be present in optimal proportions. The deficient amino acid is called the *limiting amino acid.* If a food with a limiting amino acid is combined with another food containing that limiting amino acid, protein quality is improved.

Vegetarian diets tend to lack one or another of the essential amino acids. For example, most rice is low in lysine, while some legumes are low in methionine but high in lysine. So a meal of rice and beans (legumes) provides a combination of food proteins. Nuts or seeds and legumes also provide complementary proteins.

Many cultures have made use of these dietary combinations for hundred of years without understanding amino acid metabolism—for instance, the Mexican staples of beans and rice or tortillas. The Chinese and Japanese have long mixed rice and bean curd; the East Indians mix rice and lentils. In southeastern United States, the combination of rice and black-eyed peas is common. All of these combinations provide a balanced amount of essential amino acids.

Some vegetable proteins can also be supplemented with a small amount of animal protein. The Chinese use small portions of meat or fish in stir-fried vegetables and rice dishes. Americans also use this technique with dishes such as macaroni and cheese, pizza, and even the common sandwich.

Today you can buy foods that contain sufficient proteins so that, ostensibly, you will have an abundance of amino acids from which to build the neurotransmitters in your body. However, the way you cook your food has a significant effect on its amino acid value. For example, Cornell University researchers investigated the protein, amino acid, and nitrogen content of potatoes before and after cooking.[26] Fried potato skins are an increasingly popular item in the supermarket. The researchers found that frying the skin decreased its amino acid content by 45

AMINO ACID	ADULT	INFANT	CHILD (10–12 YEARS)
Cystine	13	58	27
Histidine	16	28	20
Isoleucine	10	70	30
Leucine	14	161	45
Lysine	12	103	60
Methionine	13	58	27
Phenylalanine	14	125	27
Threonine	7	87	35
Tryptophan	3.5	17	4
Tyrosine	14	125	27
Valine	10	93	33

percent. Frying the inside of the potato, as in french frying, decreased its amino acid level by 36 percent. By contrast, baking the potato lowered the amino acid content of the skin by only 5 percent, and baking actually raised the amino acid content of the inside of the potato 13 percent. The skin of the potato has more amino acids than the inside, so you should bake your potatoes and eat the skin as well as the inside.

The above table shows the estimated daily essential amino acid requirements (given in milligrams per kilogram of body weight) based on a number of research reports.*

Can you manipulate your amino acid intake to affect your brain? You certainly can, but it is best to do it through diet rather than to dose yourself with amino acids without medical supervision. If you want to calm yourself or fall asleep more easily, eat a meal high in carbohydrates and low in protein, which will raise your brain levels of tryptophan and the neurotransmitter serotonin. Choices for a high-carbohydrate breakfast (not a balanced meal, but one weighted toward raising tryptophan) might include any of the following foods:

Pears   Pancakes with syrup
Pineapple juice   Bran muffin
Oat cereal   Decaffeinated coffee or tea
English muffin and jam

*Reprinted with permission. The Merck Manual, Chart 77—Estimated Amino Acids Requirements. 14th Edition, pg 888.

Choices for a high-carbohydrate lunch might include any of the following:

Spaghetti	Whole wheat toast and tomatoes
Macaroni	Cranberry juice
Fresh green beans	Apple pie
Rye bread	Lemon meringue pie
Potato pancakes	Decaffeinated coffee or tea, or fruit juice

Choice for a high-carbohydrate dinner might include:

Fettucini	Vegetable casserole
Baked potato stuffed with vegetables	Apricots
Barley	Cherries
Eggplant	

If you want to be stimulated, be as sharp as possible, and use your memory, or if you are going to participate in an athletic competition, you can stimulate your norepinephrine, dopamine, and acetylcholine levels by eating a diet rich in protein, especially tyrosine and lecithin (to produce acetylcholine). Choices for a high-protein breakfast might include any of the following:

Eggs	Fish
Cottage cheese	Meat
Potatoes	Milk
Yogurt	Caffeinated coffee or tea

Choices for a high-protein lunch might include:

Egg salad	Soybean products
Sliced turkey	Chili
Cheese	Tuna
Sliced chicken	Caffeinated coffee or tea

Choices for a high-protein dinner might include:

Steak	Pork chops
Lamb chops	Halibut
Veal chops	Blue fish

Chef's salad	Pizza with cheese
Salmon steaks	Milk
Cheese souffle	Caffeinated coffee or tea

The interaction in the brain among diet, amino acids, and neurotransmitters is very complicated and depends on many factors. For instance, in a paper presented at the 1987 annual meeting of the American Psychological Association, psychologist Michael Trulson questioned the immediate cause and effect of ingesting amino acids and changes in behavior.[27] Trulson described experiments in which 10 grams of tryptophan per day were given alone or with noncompeting amino acids and brain waves were checked in the area where dopamine receptors are most dense. He concluded that there was no change in electrical activity or function.

Dr. Trulson suggested that there is no "simple relationship" between diet and brain function, but that perhaps there is a "lag time."[28] He pointed out that it takes from ten days to two weeks for antidepressant medication to take effect and that perhaps there is also a delay in the effect of dietary amino acids on brain function.

The National Institute of Child Health and Human Development (NICHD) now supports research on the relationship between nutrition and behavior to further probe the intriguing but contradictory and puzzling findings of researchers thus far. As the *NICHD Guide for Researchers* points out:

> Behind the expression of all ingestive behavior lies the neurophysiology and neurochemistry of hunger and satiety. Important observations on the effect of nutrient intake on levels of cerebral neurotransmitters such as serotonin and acetylcholine have been made that pave the way for studies on the influence of diet on behavior.[29]

As scientists continue their studies, more and more information will emerge. Next to water, protein is the most abundant substance in your body. All of your cells contain protein, and you could not think without the protein in your brain. Amino acids are the building blocks of protein and, thus, of your brain, your body, and your life itself. They are extremely powerful in various combinations. If you are smart, your amino acids made you that way. Treat them with respect.

⊰ 3 ⊱

Food: Vitamins, Minerals, and Your Brain

L aura, a pretty, shy, twenty-four-year-old bank teller, developed *Tourette's syndrome, a little understood condition whose symptoms are twitching and uncontrollable utterances. Her head would jerk and she would start swearing, which frightened her co-workers and customers. She was given* haloperidol, *a drug that dampens the production of dopamine, a brain neurotransmitter involved with movement and stress. The drug stopped the symptoms, but it affected Laura's ability to think, to the point where she could no longer cash checks correctly. The situation was even more frustrating because she had been in line to be promoted; instead, she was fired.*

Many physicians tried, but none could help her. Finally, a young doctor suggested she take large doses of nicotinic acid, *or vitamin B_3. The B vitamins are known to affect the central nervous system. A severe B_3 deficiency, called* pellagra, *causes mental abberations including excitement, disorientation, memory impairment, confusion, and delirium.[1] Laura's symptoms cleared within a month, and within two months she was rehired at her old job.*

Unfortunately, after five months on B_3, Laura developed symptoms of nausea, fatigue, and yellowed skin. She had developed a chemical hepatitis, a liver problem caused by the massive doses of B_3. She was hospitalized, taken off the vitamin, detoxified, and then returned home. Several days later, her Tourette's syndrome returned, and she was again dismissed from her job.

In desperation, Laura's mother telephoned Herman Baker, Ph.D., director of the Division of Nutrition and Metabolism at the Newark site of New Jersey Medical School's and a professor of preventive medicine. Dr.

29

Baker, a world famous authority on vitamin research, suggested to Laura's physician that perhaps B₃, but in a smaller dose, should be tried. The Tourette symptoms cleared, the liver problems did not return, and Laura is now employed at another bank.[2]

Dr. Baker explains that B₃ is not a conventional treatment for Tourette's syndrome; nor has it been tested as such, but it seemed to work for that young woman.

In another dramatic case involving a B vitamin, an eighty-one-year-old man, Mr. L., was admitted to a western hospital with a one-week history of irritable mood associated with hyperactivity, sleeplessness, grand delusions, sexual indiscretion, and reckless and agitated behavior. He felt his home town was planning a day of celebration in his honor to which several Hollywood personalities were invited. He was so active, in fact, that six younger men were required to restrain him at the time of admission to the hospital. Mr. L. had no family history of mental illness. His test results were normal and he had not been taking medicines. The only test that came back abnormal was the test for vitamin B₁₂ levels in his blood.

Mr. L. received a daily dose of vitamin B₁₂ in his muscle while he was in the hospital, then monthly injections after discharge.

The supplemental B₁₂ returned Mr. L. to a normal mental state, and six months later he was still completely normal. This case supports other recent reports that psychiatric symptoms may antedate other major clinical manifestations of B₁₂ deficiency such as pernicious anemia.[3]

There is much about vitamins that is yet unknown and untested. They are by no means always harmless, as demonstrated by Laura's experience. For nearly half a century, researchers have been trying to determine the complex ways in which vitamins and minerals interact with each other and with the other nutrients and elements. There are more than forty chemical elements and compounds in your body that must follow a predetermined recipe to keep you "cooking" just right, physically and mentally. These substances are found in the vitamins, minerals, fats, proteins, and carbohydrates that are essential to your brain and body functions. Vitamins are the team players who work with the other substances to convert the food you eat into energy and tissue growth. They help repair damage, maintain immunity, and other important processes.

Minerals perform a variety of functions, including influencing the acid/base balance of your body fluids and the distribution of water throughout your body. They also play an essential role in the formation of bones and teeth and in the life processes of your cells. Vitamins and minerals are exquisitely measured; too much or too little of any one of them can throw your system off track.

What amounts of vitamins and minerals do you need? The Food and Nutrition Board of the National Academy of Sciences periodically issues recommended dietary allowances (RDA's). The values given are estimates based on a review of the current nutrition literature and, hence, subject to controversy. In fact, when they met in 1985, there was so much debate among the members of the board that they could not agree, and consequently no new RDA's were issued. This happened despite, or perhaps because of, the new developments in nutritional science since the last RDA's were issued in 1980.[4]

The RDA's are supposedly set at levels high enough to prevent classic deficiency symptoms such as the skin eruptions and mental disorders associated with pellagra. However, preventing classic deficiencies may be just one of the important functions of vitamins. The complete role of nutrients in your health is far more complex, involving a multitude of biochemical reactions, many of which are still mysterious, in your cells.

For certain vitamins and minerals, RDA's have not even been set because there is not enough knowledge on which to base them. Instead, "estimated safe and adequate dietary allowances" have been designated.[5]

While a description of the research on vitamins alone could fill many volumes, in this book we are primarily concerned with the known and suspected effects of these nutrients on brain function.

The effects of a vitamin or mineral deficiency can be unrecognized, and when the missing nutrient is added, its benefits can be dramatic. Dr. Baker, for example, diagnosed a genetic condition, biotin dependency, in 1985. He was sent blood samples from a newborn who was having almost continuous convulsions. He found a deficiency of the B vitamin *biotin* and suggested that the pediatrician give the baby 75 micrograms of the vitamin. The baby's seizures continued. Dr. Baker then suggested increasing the dosage to 10 milligrams which is a massive dose. After the new dosage was administered, the seizures stopped. The baby thrived because the high dose of biotin overcame a metabolic deficit.

When the baby was three years old, the pediatrician decided that perhaps the seizure cessation was just coincidental to the biotin supplement, and he told the mother to stop giving it to the child. Within a short time, the toddler again began to have convulsions.[6]

Dr. Baker, an enthusiastic, cigar-smoking, no-nonsense type of man, believes that many current testing methods do not accurately detect vitamin levels, particularly as far as B_{12} is concerned. He points out that using radioactive tracers, or radioimmunoassay tests, to detect the level of B_{12} in the blood does not produce an accurate measure, because tracers count an inactive form of B_{12}, which cannot be used by the human body, as well as the active form of B_{12}, which can. The FDA agrees with Dr. Baker's argument. Instead of the radioimmunoassay test, Dr. Baker employs a test involving micro-animals *(protozoa)* that process B_{12} the same way humans do.[7] Vitamin B_{12}, which can be obtained only from meat, dairy products, and eggs, is vital to the growth and maintenance of a healthy brain and nervous system.

Dr. Baker believes there are other undetected vitamin deficiencies that contribute to subtle behavior effects that are escaping detection by the usual methods of physical examination. "Classical deficiency diseases have all but disappeared in the United States because of improved nutritional knowledge and the enrichment of certain foods," he maintains, "but marginal or subclinical stages of vitamin deficiency certainly do exist."[8] In a 1967–68 study of 674 New York City schoolchildren between the ages of ten and thirteen years, he found that 25 percent had undetected marginal deficiencies that can affect their intellectual performance.[9]

MARGINAL DEFICIENCY

Marginal deficiency, by definition, is a state of gradual vitamin depletion in which there is evidence of personal lack of well-being associated with impairment of certain chemical reactions in the body.[10] The reactions impaired are those that depend on sufficient amounts of vitamins.

Vitamin deficiency is not something that occurs abruptly or acutely. During the *preliminary stage,* body stores of a micronutrient are gradually depleted. When there is not enough of a particular vitamin to work for the body, the body's chemistry is impaired. In this preliminary stage, there is *no indication* of depletion in clinical terms of growth or appearance.

The next degree of depletion is called the *physiological* stage. These changes are ones that you might not associate with nutrient deficiencies—for example, loss of appetite, depression, irritability, anxiety, insomnia, or sleepiness. The person is not sufficiently ill to seek medical care or go to the hospital, yet his or her general health is less than optimal.

If the deficiency continues, symptoms of classic deficiency disease will appear. This is called the *clinical stage*. Left untreated, it is followed by the *anatomical stage,* in which death will occur without nutritional intervention.[11]

Marginal deficiencies, since they are so subtle, are difficult to identify. Only in recent years has sufficient evidence accumulated to call attention to this gray area of nutrition.

To demonstrate just how the stages of a vitamin deficiency occur, a former research assistant of Dr. Baker's placed himself on a diet deficient in folic acid (vitamin B complex).[12] That meant no green vegetables, beans, walnuts, or chicken liver, all good sources of the vitamin necessary for the manufacture of genetic material (DNA) and healthy red blood cells. Two and a half weeks after he began the diet, he noticed a low level of folic acid in his blood. After ten to twelve weeks, he began to detect a biochemical sign—an abnormal waste product of metabolism in his urine. Sixteen weeks into the diet, a bone marrow examination was performed to see whether he had any signs of anemia and cell changes. He began to see evidence of folic acid deficiency in his red blood cells. Some seventeen weeks later, his body's new red blood cells were being formed with low folic acid. It was at that point—twenty-five weeks after beginning the diet—that he saw the full-blown anemia due to folic acid deficiency. Dr. Baker maintains that

a clinician who looks at a blood picture and sees a patient suffering from an early, *marginal* deficiency, as in the case above when the research assistant first had low levels of folic acid, should treat that patient then, rather than wait for the *clinical* signs. In the case of folic acid deficiency, it took twenty-five to thirty weeks to show a full-blown anemia. Many clinicians, however, would just ignore these early signs. They would say vitamins are ubiquitous and there is no need for supplementation. However, if there were a similar picture as the research assistant's but instead of folic acid deficiency there was too much sugar in the blood, what would a physician do? He'd say, "Hey, I'm not going to wait around till this fellow goes blind and his kidneys fail," as can happen with advanced diabetes. He would begin to treat him with insulin. He wouldn't wait.[13]

Only a blood analysis of vitamins can help detect sub-clinical deficits and can avoid physiologic and eventually full-blown vitamin deficits, the same as one would do to check cholesterol levels to avoid eventual heart disease.

According to Dr. Baker, many older persons suffer from undiagnosed marginal deficiencies that cause mental and physical problems. They have these nutrient deficiencies, even though they may be eating nutritious meals and taking supplemental vitamins orally, because they can no longer absorb sufficient nutrients. He and his colleagues proved this by testing the elderly residents.

We found that the residents' livers were not able to bind enough vitamins as younger people can and that the residents were also taking drugs that deplete nutrients. Since they could not absorb sufficient vitamins from food or supplementation by mouth to saturate the liver, we gave them an injection of a bolus of vitamins, more than the conventional RDA's. We continued to monitor them and found their vitamin levels were normal for three months; then began to decline after that until they were back to deficient after a year. Therefore, we felt they needed vitamin injections every three months.

The nurses told us the patients improved following the injection. Some who were bedridden were able to get out of bed. Others were able to return to a sheltered workshop. All seemed to function better mentally. In fact, the nurses asked us if we wouldn't give them vitamin injections, too.[14]

Dr. Baker feels that many clinicians are unaware that widespread subclinical or marginal vitamin deficiencies exist and do not know how to test for these deficiencies. However, Dr. Baker has developed vitamin testing procedures for all twelve vitamins. The vitamin tests are now available for defining hidden and overt vitamin deficits and have appeared in many medical journals.[15]

"Get a blood vitamin profile and don't guess about your vitamin health," says Dr. Baker. "You get a blood sugar not to guess about diabetes. Why not do the same for vitamins?"

Paul Lachance, Ph.D., a food science professor at Rutgers University and one of the creators of the diets for astronauts in space, also believes that widespread marginal deficiencies exist, particularly among the forty million Americans who go on weight-loss regimens each year.[16]

Dr. Lachance was one of the experts who studied eleven of the most popular reducing diets and found that not one regimen contained all of the RDA's for the thirteen nutrients studied.[17] As Dr. Lachance points out, "You can't go below 1200 calories a day and still meet all these needs. It's difficult to assure nutritional adequacy with less than 1,800 to 2,000 calories."[18]

If you eat a diet meal accompanied by a cocktail or a glass of wine, you may deplete your nutrient levels even more. Alcohol, as discussed later in this chapter, depletes vitamins. Smoke a cigarette, and you will deplete your nutrients even more.

Dr. Lachance believes that pollution and food processing are not taken into account as depleters of vitamins. He believes that vitamins C and A are depleted by pollutants in the environment. He also feels that marginal deficiencies in vitamin B_6 are widespread and that bread should be supplemented with the vitamin. "We are not asking them to add additional B_6 to bread—just to replace what has been lost through processing," he explains.[19]

All right, suppose you do have a subclinical vitamin deficiency. What does that mean, physically and mentally? Says Dr. Baker,

> You'll always feel tired. You may have insomnia and/or a loss of appetite. A decreased ability to concentrate. Your brain does not function well. You complain to your physician, "I feel under the weather. I don't know what is bothering me but I keep getting colds." The doctor examines you and tells you he can find nothing wrong. So he says, "Take some vitamins!" If you have an absorption problem or the liver cannot bind or store vitamins, you can take a ton of vitamins but you will just enrich the sewage system.
>
> You can take one-tenth or three-tenths [of a milligram of] vitamin B_1 and you won't absorb anymore than one-tenth milligram since that is all your body can absorb at one time. The rest is wasted. But if you break the dose into three times a day, you can absorb a total of three-tenths of a milligram of thiamin a day.[20]

According to Dr. Baker, taking vitamins with food will aid absorption, while mineral supplements are best absorbed when taken between meals. "Not only lay persons but physicians are often unaware of these simple facts," he maintains.[21]

Since the brain and body cannot be disconnected, the following are descriptions of the known and proposed potential effects of vitamins and minerals on both your body and brain function:

Vitamin A. The nutritional requirement for the fat-soluble vitamin A for you, as an individual, will depend on a number of related factors, including age, growth rate, sex, your body's efficiency in absorbing and storing the vitamin, and the efficiency of transporting it in your blood and utilizing it by your cells. Intestinal, kidney, and liver disease tend to increase the need for vitamin A. Other vitamin A depleters include alcohol, cortisone (often used to treat inflammation), and mineral oil (taken frequently, especially by older people, in laxatives). Vitamin A is needed for the health of the skin and the inner lining of the body—the mucous membranes that protect the throat, nasal passages, bronchial tubes, digestive system, and genitourinary tract. It helps to maintain the structure of cell membranes and is necessary for the healthy functioning of your immune system. Vitamin A is also needed for the maintenance and growth of teeth, hair, bones, and glands. It is vital for vision. A vitamin A deficiency can also affect how iron is used by your body.

A government survey showed that half of the people aged eighteen to forty-four years in the United States take in less than the RDA of vitamin A.[22] The RDA is 5,000 international units for men, 4,000 international units for women, and 1,400 to 3,000 international units for infants and children.

Overdosing on vitamin A can cause drowsiness, irritability, headache, and vomiting. It can cause pressure on the brain that produces tumorlike symptoms. Overdosing on beta-carotene, the vegetable form of vitamin A, does not produce the serious side effects of a vitamin A overdose but may cause your skin to turn yellow.[23]

Vitamin A exists in two main forms in nature—as *retinol,* found only in animal sources, and as certain *carotenoids,* found mainly in yellow vegetables and fruit. Carotenoids are only one-third as potent as retinol. High levels of vitamin E can block the conversion of beta-carotene into vitamin A.

Vitamin B$_1$ *(thiamine).* The link between vitamin B$_1$ and brain function is direct and strong. Our bodies cannot manufacture vitamin B$_1$, yet it is needed to process the only fuel the brain can use: glucose. Because of

VITAMIN A SOURCES

VERY GOOD	GOOD
Beef liver	Milk
Bok choy	Prunes
Spinach	Asparagus
Cantaloupe	Green beans
Kale	Brussels sprouts
Carrots	Corn
Broccoli	Eggs
Apricots	Orange, tomato, or
Red peppers	grapefruit juice
Fish oil	Margarine
Sweet potatoes	Peas
Butternut squash	Yogurt
Papaya	Peaches

this vital need in thiamine-dependent carbohydrate metabolism, the nervous system is particularly susceptible to thiamine deficiency.[24] Vitamin B$_1$ is necessary not only for the health of your nerve tissue, but also for your intestinal and cardiovascular function, appetite, and growth. Deficiency in its early stages produces fatigue, irritation, poor memory, sleep disturbance, chest pain, loss of appetite, abdominal discomfort, and constipation. Later the symptoms progress to numbness, a burning sensation in the feet, calf muscle cramps, and leg pains.

Primary deficiency of vitamin A, of course, occurs from inadequate intake. Secondary deficiency arises from an increased requirement due to an overactive thyroid gland, pregnancy, breast feeding, or fever. It also results from impaired absorption, as in chronic diarrhea, and from inadequate utilization, as in severe liver disease.

A combination of decreased intake, impaired absorption, inadequate utilization, and increased requirements occur in alcoholism. Even a glass of wine or a cocktail reduces absorption of thiamine by your gut. Incidently, marinating meat in wine, soy sauce, or vinegar depletes between 50 and 75 percent of its thiamine content.

Thiamine treatment—as much as 300 milligrams per day—is used in cases of Wernicke's encephalopathy, an acute brain disorder sometimes called "cerebral beriberi" in which, in the early stages, there is mental confusion, inability to think of a word, and making up of "facts." As it progresses, there are delusions, loss of memory, loss of balance, and eye problems. This syndrome is associated with thiamine deficiency. In industrialized countries, the disorder occurs most frequently in alcoholics. In fact, the brain damage caused by alcohol in this syndrome has only recently been directly attributed to a lack of thiamine. Australian psychiatrists, as a result, want to add thiamine to alcoholic beverages—beer, in particular—to prevent brain damage. They calculated that the annual cost of adding thiamine to the entire supply of Australian beer would be no higher than the cost of supporting eight alcoholics with Wernicke's psychosis for one year.[25] Many other Australian researchers believe that treatment with thiamine and abstinence from alcohol can reverse brain damage, including the shrinkage, caused by alcohol.[26] Cerebral beriberi has sometimes also been associated with intravenous feedings, starvation, neurological disease, chronic infection, kidney dialysis, cancer, anemia, and scurvy.[27]

What about marginal deficiency? As early as 1946, one scientist observed that a liberal thiamine intake improved a number of mental and physical skills of children in orphanages.[28]

In a study concerning human starvation, one researcher observed thiamine deficiency in close detail and found that lack of well-being, anxiety, hysteria, nausea, depression, and loss of appetite preceded any aspect of the clinical state of beriberi. These personality changes were all typical of pure thiamine deficiency and were normalized within a short period following the addition of thiamine to the diet.[29]

Other studies, using a behavior test called the Minnesota Multiphasic Personality Index (MMPI), have demonstrated that adverse behavioral changes precede physical findings in thiamine deficiency, as shown in Mr. L.'s case at the beginning of this chapter, as well as in deficiencies of vitamin C and riboflavin. The deficiencies of these nutrients were induced in human subjects under carefully controlled laboratory conditions; then subjects were given the MMPI test. Hypochondria, depression, hysteria, and, in some cases, manic and crazy behavior were described by the investigators as occurring before any specific physical signs of vitamin deficiency were observed.[30]

Extensive studies on the effects of thiamine depletion on humans red blood cells have definitely been correlated with changes in behavior.[31] Depleted subjects most commonly complained of lethargy, loss of appetite, and fatigue. Since no obvious physical signs of thiamine deficiency were noted, such symptoms were believed to be caused by marginal B_1 deficiency. This belief was proven true when the behavior of subjects reverted to normal within two to three days after thiamine was again present in their diets.[32]

A group of enzymes called *thiaminases,* which destroy thiamine, have been found in raw fish (as in an increasingly popular Japanese dish, sushi), shellfish, some berries, brussels sprouts, and red cabbage. However, these enzymes are inactivated by cooking.

The RDA's for thiamine are 1.5 milligrams for adults and 0.3 to 1.1 milligrams for infants and children.

VITAMIN B_1 SOURCES	
VERY GOOD	GOOD
Wheat germ	Collard greens
Lobster	Enriched or
Pinto beans	whole-wheat spaghetti
Roast pork	Enriched or brown rice
Kasha	Fortified milk
Oat flakes	Asparagus
Sunflower seeds	Lima beans
Brewer's yeast	Cauliflower
Soybeans	Pecans
Black-eyed peas	Shredded wheat
Green peas	Broccoli
	Whole-wheat bread

Vitamin B_2 *(riboflavin).* Vitamin B_2 is also called *lactoflavin* or *hepatoflavin* because milk and liver are its main natural sources. Deficiency is associated with skin diseases, including pellagra, and with lip and mouth lesions. The result could be teary, bloodshot eyes or indigestion, since B_2 aids in the digestion of fats. Cracks around the mouth and flaky skin around the nose, eyebrows and hair line are also signs of B_2 deficiency. Easy fatigability and irritability are also signs. This vitamin is believed to fight stress. Riboflavin has a high affinity for your brain and helps to explain the long-standing observation that even in severe riboflavin deficiency, its concentration in the brain does not decline appreciably.

Ironically, while riboflavin reportedly fights stress and is similar in chemical structure to chlorpromazine, the tranquilizer Thorazine, chlorpromazine depletes riboflavin. Inhibition of riboflavin metabolism is also observed with the tricyclic antidepressant drugs imipramine and amitriptyline.[33]

The RDA's for vitamin B_2 are 1.7 milligrams for men, 1.2 to 1.3 milligrams for women, and 0.4 to 1.6 milligrams for infants and children.

VITAMIN B_2 SOURCES

VERY GOOD	GOOD
Beef and beef liver	Noodles
Milk	Peas
Brewer's yeast	Spinach
Ham	Puffed and flaked wheat
Sunflower seeds	Chocolate chip cookies
Broccoli	Oatmeal with raisins
Butternut squash	Custard
Wild rice	Asparagus
Almonds	
Cottage cheese	

Vitamin B_3 (*niacin, niacinamide,* or *nicotinic acid*). At least forty biochemical reactions depend on niacin. Perhaps the most important involves red blood cells, which carry oxygen to all parts of your body, including your brain. Niacin, when taken in large doses, causes flushing, itching, dilation of the blood vessels, increased blood flow in the brain, and decreased blood pressure. It can lower blood cholesterol and is being used for that purpose. Niacin also has been found to counteract some of the effects of caffeine (see page 148).

Niacin is made in your gut from the amino acid tryptophan, which derives from protein. Tryptophan also serves as the raw material for the manufacture of the calming neurotransmitter serotonin. Therefore, it is not surprising that striking and profound mental disturbance may frequently occur as part of a vitamin B_3 deficiency. The brain and nerve symptoms caused by B_3 deficiency are not completely understood, but problems with serotonin have been suggested as the basis of psychosis that occurs in the B_3 deficiency disease pellagra. Also suspect is dietary excess of the amino acid leucine, which causes symptoms similar to pellagra and impairs serotonin utilization.[34]

Large doses of B_3 in the form of niacin have been used to treat schizophrenia. Drs. Abram Hoffer and Humphry Osmond, who consider the disease to be caused by a biochemical abnormality, reported outstanding improvement in many of the thousands of patients treated with B_3. But other investigators reported that they could not duplicate those results. There is a theory that schizophrenia is actually many diseases, some of which are responsive to B_3. This seems to be backed by a study made by Dr. J. Richard Wittenborn of Rutgers University. Dr. Wittenborn studied schizophrenics for two years at a New Jersey state hospital. At first he found that patients receiving the vitamin showed no impressive gains as compared to patients not receiving it. But when Dr. Wittenborn went back over the original study, he decided that some patients treated with the vitamin had responded more than others and that the response was significant.[35]

Usually, not enough B_3 is manufactured from tryptophan by bacteria in your gut to keep you in good health. You need to obtain more of it

VITAMIN B_3 SOURCES	
VERY GOOD	GOOD
Turkey	Muffins made with enriched
Tofu	flour
Calf's liver	Enriched or whole-wheat noodles
Bulgur wheat	Oats
Puffed wheat	Corn flakes
Halibut	Barley
Peanuts	Kale
Hamburger	Broccoli
Tuna	Enriched French bread
Coffee	Bagels
Cottage cheese	Peanuts
Peas	Brown rice
Beans	Mangos
	Milk

from your diet. Men need 16 to 19 milligrams, women need 13 to 14 milligrams, and infants and children need 6 to 16 milligrams.

Vitamin B$_6$ *(pyridoxine).* Vitamin B$_6$ is believed to act as a partner for more than one hundred different enzymes. A number of the neurotransmitters depend on B$_6$ for formation. A deficiency in this vitamin is known to cause depression and mental confusion. The occurrence of seizures in experimental animals in response to vitamin B$_6$ antagonists has been observed by many. Similar seizures were observed in human infants made vitamin B$_6$ deficient intentionally or inadvertently when they were fed a commercial infant formula in which the vitamin had not been properly preserved. Certain substances that deplete B$_6$ also produce deficiency seizures.[36]

Vitamin B$_6$ also reportedly helps rid the body tissues of the excess fluid that causes some of the symptoms of premenstrual tension.

Two possible causes have been suggested for the frequent deficiency of vitamin B$_6$ in alcoholics. Alcohol may inhibit the body's absorption of the vitamin from the intestine and it may cause B$_6$ to break down prematurely in the blood. Reduced levels of vitamin B$_6$ have also been found in smokers, but this may be due to their higher alcohol use.

Estrogen and cortisone deplete B$_6$. Storage over a long period of time

VITAMIN B$_6$ SOURCES	
VERY GOOD	GOOD
Wheat Germ	Brown rice
Brewer's yeast	Ham
Bananas	Spinach
Fish	Peanuts
Soybeans	Cantaloupe
Tomatoes	Milk
Salmon	Cabbage
Kale	Raisins
Spinach	Broccoli
Beans	Asparagus
	Sunflower seeds
	Cauliflower

diminishes the vitamin. Freezing vegetables results in 57 to 77 percent reduction of their B_6 content.

Overdosing on B_6, on the other hand, is very unwise. A study reported in the *New England Journal of Medicine* in 1983 reported the loss of balance and numbness suffered by seven young adults who took from 2 to 6 grams of pyridoxine daily for several months to a year.[37] Discontinuation of the supplements resulted in improvement in all subjects, although a few continued to have residual abnormalities in nerve conduction as late as six months afterward.

The RDA's for vitamin B_6 are 2.2 milligrams for men, 2 milligrams for women, and 0.3 to 1.6 milligrams for infants and children.

Vitamin B_{12}. Vitamin B_{12} is needed for normal growth, a healthy nervous system, and normal red blood cell formation. It can be found only in animal and dairy products. A B_{12} deficiency produces pernicious anemia, a severe anemia similar to that caused by a B_6 deficiency. Vitamin B_{12} anemia is rarely the result of dietary deficiency, except in vegans (vegetarians who consume no animal food or dairy products), since the liver stores sufficient quantities to sustain the body's needs for three to five years. The inability to absorb this vitamin is the major cause of pernicious anemia, which can lead to brain and nerve damage. In most patients, the symptoms develop insidiously and progressively as the large liver stores of B_{12} are depleted. Symptoms include loss of appetite, intermittent constipation and diarrhea, and stomach pain. A deficiency produces patchy, diffuse, and progressive nerve degeneration. There may be

VITAMIN B_{12} SOURCES	
VERY GOOD	GOOD
Beef liver	Swiss cheese
Roast beef	Whole or skim milk
Ham	Eggs
Fillet of sole	Cottage cheese
Oysters	Yogurt
Sardines	
Crab	
Herring	

a loss of balance, numbness and weakness of the limbs irritability, mild depression, or paranoia, a condition known as megaloblastic madness.[38]

Alcohol, estrogen, and sleeping pills can lower B_{12} levels in the body. Vitamin C, however, does not destroy vitamin B_{12}, as some medical reports have proposed. Dr. Baker and associates tested Nobelist Linus Pauling, an advocate of massive doses of vitamin C, and Pauling's colleagues, all of whom had taken large amounts of vitamin C for years. Dr. Baker found that all of the vitamin C takers had normal levels of B_{12}.[39]

The RDA's for B_{12} are 3 micrograms for adults and 0.5 to 3 micrograms for infants and children.

Folic acid *(folacin, or folate).* Folic acid, a vitamin of the B complex, is necessary for the division and replacement of red blood cells. It is needed for protein metabolism and the utilization of sugar. A deficiency anemia may occur, especially in menstruating women, but it is less common than other anemias caused by a B_3 deficiency. Folic acid is needed in the manufacture of genetic material. A deficiency can also cause gastrointestinal upsets and emotional irritability.

Alcohol and contraceptives reduce the body's absorption of this vitamin and thus increase the risk of deficiency. Sunlight and aspirin can deplete it. Folic acid supplementation has been used in the treatment of alcohol withdrawal. The sugar from fruit, vegetables, and grain enhances the absorption of folic acid.

FOLIC ACID SOURCES

VERY GOOD	GOOD
Deep-green leafy vegetables	Cantaloupe
Carrots	Dark rye flour
Apricots	Shredded wheat
Asparagus	Cottage cheese
Navy beans	Chuck pot roast
Chicken liver	Avocados
Wheat bran	Eggs
Walnuts	Sweet potatoes
Brewer's yeast	Grapefruit juice
Beans, especially soybeans	
Orange juice	

The RDA for folic acid is 400 micrograms for adults and 30 to 300 micrograms for infants and children.

Biotin. Biotin is a B vitamin involved in many of your body's functions, including the metabolism of sugar and the formation of certain fatty acids. It was once thought that biotin deficiencies occur only in infants. However, in a 1942 study, seven adult volunteers were fed 200 grams of dehydrated egg whites per day, in addition to an otherwise balanced diet.[40] (A vitamin antagonist in raw eggs contains *avidin,* a substance that binds up biotin and makes it nonabsorbable; cooking destroys the avidin.) After five weeks, the subjects displayed symptoms of mild depression, lassitude, sleepiness, hallucinations, anxiety with muscle pain, and oversensitivity to pain stimuli. After eight weeks, loss of appetite, a grayish pallor, and a skin rash occurred. The experiment was terminated because of the falling food intake. The symptoms disappeared within five days of treatment with 75 to 300 milligrams per day of intravenous biotin.

A biotin deficiency is rare, except in children born with an inborn error of metabolism.

The safe and adequate intake for adults is 100 to 200 micrograms. Infants and children need 35 to 85 micrograms.

BIOTIN SOURCES	
VERY GOOD	GOOD
Peanuts	Chicken
Liver	Halibut
Mushrooms	Cauliflower
Yeast	

Pantothenic acid. Pantothenic acid is needed for the adrenal glands, which are located above the kidneys and which secrete adrenaline, and to convert fat and glucose into energy. In studies with both rats and humans, those with high levels of pantothenic acid had more endurance when swimming in cold water.[41] The rats with low levels of the vitamin were able to swim only sixteen minutes in the cold water, while those with high levels were able to swim sixty-two minutes. The humans with high levels of the vitamin showed less wear and tear on a biochemical level than did those with low levels during a ten-minute swim in forty-five-degree water.

Some researchers believe that when the adrenal glands contain high levels of pantothenic acid, the body is better able to deal with stress.[42] In fact, the discoverer of pantothenic acid, Dr. Roger Williams, named it the Latin word for "from all sides."

Pantothenic acid deficiency is rare, because the vitamin is found in most foods. However, food processing such as canning or freezing destroys as much as 75 percent of a food's pantothenic acid content. Sleeping pills, alcohol, caffeine, and estrogen also destroy it. A deficiency may result in such symptoms as malaise, abdominal distress, and a burning sensation in the feet associated with numbness.[43]

The safe and effective dietary dose is 4 to 7 milligrams daily for adults, 35–40 nanograms for infants, and 65–120 nanograms for children and adolescents.

PANTOTHENIC ACID SOURCES	
VERY GOOD	GOOD
Brewer's yeast	Eggs
Beef liver	Milk
Bran	Fresh vegetables
Cereal	

Vitamin C *(ascorbic acid).* The level of vitamin C in the brain is second only to that found in the adrenal glands. This has led researchers to believe that vitamin C plays an important role in fighting stress. Since vitamin C is so abundant in the brain, it is assumed to be needed there, but its full role has yet to be identified. The interplay between vitamin C and the amino acids, the building blocks of protein, suggests that vitamin C may play a vital role in the regulation of neurotransmitters. Vitamin C has been found to be needed as a helper in the manufacture of norepinephrine, a major brain neurotransmitter that acts as a stimulant (see chapter 11).[44] Numerous studies have noted a relationship between vitamin C, brain function, and behavior.[45]

Behavior such as smoking and drinking alcoholic beverages may be

VITAMIN C SOURCES

VERY GOOD	GOOD
Brussels sprouts	Enriched flour
Cauliflower	Tomatoes
Freshly squeezed orange juice	Puffed wheat
Sweet potatoes	Waffles
Broccoli	Potatoes
Papaya	Collard greens
Cabbage	Spinach
Watermelon	Apricots
Grapefruit	Avocados
Green and red peppers	Pineapple
Honeydew melon	Corn flakes
Strawberries	
Kale	

made a little less harmful by vitamin C. This is because vitamin C helps prevent damage from free radicals, the extremely reactive, unstable molecules that are produced in the body through normal biological processes as well as in the environment through radiation, sunlight, air pollution, cigarette smoke, and other chemical processes. Free radicals have been linked to aging, cancer, arthritis, lung inflammation, and senility. (See pages 195 and 199 for more about free radicals.)

In laboratory experiments, it has been shown that vitamin C inhibits the growth of cancerous tumor cells and is potentially toxic to skin cancer cells. Vitamin C can block the formation of *nitrosamine,* a class of chemical compounds, many of which are known to cause cancer in laboratory animals. In addition, vitamin C has been shown to bind with lead, thereby lowering the level of harmful lead in the body. Lead damages the brain, particularly in children. Smokers should pay particular heed to these protective properties of vitamin C, because the cigarette smoke they consume contains large amounts of free radicals, nitrates (a chemical precursor of nitrosamine), and other known and suspected cancer-causing agents, as well as lead. This may explain why, on average, heavy smokers are known to have lower levels of vitamin C in their blood than do nonsmokers.

Vitamin C is also needed for teeth and bone formation, bone fracture healing, wound and burn healing, and resistance to infections and other diseases. A deficiency can produce weakness, swollen and tender joints, loose teeth, delayed wound healing, easy bruising, and loss of appetite.

Vitamin C is reduced by aspirin. Cooking can destroy a food's vitamin C content.

The RDA's for vitamin C is 60 milligrams for adults and 35 to 45 milligrams for children.

Vitamin D *(calciferol).* Vitamin D is needed to absorb calcium, the building block of bone, so a deficiency of this vitamin will cause rickets and other bone diseases. Alcohol may impair the body's processing of vitamin D, causing it to build up to dangerous levels. Too much vitamin D can cause loss of appetite, elevated cholesterol, drowsiness, headache, kidney failure, and calcium deposits in organs.[46]

Most of the natural foodstuffs we consume contain only trivial quantities of vitamin D. Because these small amounts appear to have little effect on the status of vitamin D in our bodies, researchers believe that there are several means by which the body obtains it, one of which is through the action of sunshine on the skin. Conversion of vitamin D to its active forms involves the liver and kidneys, both of which may become less efficient with aging.

The RDA for vitamin D is 400 international units for adults and for children.

VITAMIN D SOURCES	
VERY GOOD	GOOD
Cod liver oil	Fortified milk
Sardines	Fortified soybean milk
Salmon	Cheese
Egg yolk	
Tuna	

Vitamin E *(tocopherol).* Vitamin E is needed for healthy heart and skeletal muscles and helps to fight the effects of pollutants. Some studies suggest that dietary supplements of this vitamin may provide protection against tissue damage caused by smoking. Normally, the body helps protect itself from pollutants and other threats by the action of dietary antioxidants such as vitamins A, C, and E and *selenium*. If your diet is deficient in these, your immune system may be affected. Like vitamin C, vitamin E helps block the formation of nitrosamine. Vitamins E and C collaborate in protecting the blood vessels and other tissues against damage by oxidation. They slow down the process of deterioration of the brain and body and help prevent strokes and heart attacks. In fact, in 1987, researchers at the University of Rochester and the University of Medicine and Dentistry of New Jersey began a project with eight hundred Parkinson's patients to test vitamin E alone and in combination with an MAO-inhibitor drug because there was some indication that the vitamin works to slow the progression of the disease.[47]

Heat and freezing destroy vitamin E.

The RDA's for vitamin E are 8 to 10 international units for men, 12 international units for women, and 3 to 7 international units for infants and children.

VITAMIN E SOURCES	
VERY GOOD	GOOD
Walnuts	Coconut
Almonds	Olive oil
Sunflower seeds	Pears
Wheat germ	Peanuts
Whole wheat	Filberts
Oils: corn, peanut,	Broccoli
safflower, sesame,	Brussels sprouts
soybean, sunflower,	Blackberries
walnut, cod liver, and	Apples
wheat germ	
Sweet potatoes	
Leeks	
Spinach	
Asparagus	
Beet greens	
Margarine	

MINERALS FOR THE MIND

Minerals perform a variety of functions in your body. There are two classes of minerals: *macronutrients* and *micronutrients.* Your body contains more of the macronutrients—magnesium, sodium, potassium and chloride—and you require more of them in your diet. The amounts range from hundreds of milligrams to grams.

The micronutrients include iron, manganese, copper, iodine, zinc, fluoride, selenium, molybdenum, chromium, aluminum, boron, nickel, silicon, and vanadium. Micronutrients, also called trace elements, are found in tiny amounts—so small they are often measured in micrograms. Your body contains some trace elements even though there is no known need for them. These include aluminum, antimony, barium, boron, bromine, gallium, germanium, gold, lithium, mercury, silver, strontium, and titanium.

Lithium, a light metal that exists in the earth's crust, has been used as a medicine since ancient Greece, when it was prescribed for gout, rheumatism, and kidney stones. Small amounts of the salts of lithium are being used to treat manic-depressive psychosis, which is characterized by wide swings between deep depression and overexcitement. Lithium has also been reported to cause alcoholics to lose their taste for liquor.[48] Exactly why it works in either case is unknown.

The Food and Nutrition Board has not determined RDA's for nineteen of the twenty-five minerals known to be in the human diet. RDA's, as mentioned, are established by the board only after it has enough scientific data to support the recommended intakes, and the board believes there are adequate data only for calcium, iron, phosphorous, iodine, magnesium, and zinc. For sodium, potassium, copper, manganese, fluoride, chromium, selenium, and molybdenum, the board has established what it calls "estimated safe and adequate daily dietary intakes" (SDI's). For the eleven remaining minerals, there is not even enough data to set SDI's.

Vitamins are organic and minerals are inorganic. Minerals, however, are generally dependent on organic molecules for transport, storage, and actual function. This characteristic binding pattern can lead to problems if high amounts of some nonessential and essential elements are present in the diet. Like vitamins, much remains unknown about how the minerals in your food and water affect your brain. The following are minerals that are known to play an important role in your brain function and general health. Sodium, chloride, and aluminum are not listed as they will be discussed in detail in later chapters (see pages 91–96 and 140–143, respectively).

Calcium. Calcium is the most abundant mineral in your body. You need it for blood clotting, the development of normal nerve tissue, regular heart beat, iron metabolism, and healthy teeth and bones. The level of calcium in blood plasma is remarkably constant at concentrations of about 10 milligrams per deciliter. Calcium within the cells is also tightly controlled. Calcium is absorbed from the intestine by a process requiring vitamin D. Milk sugar (lactose) and vitamin D can both increase calcium absorption, which is why milk and milk-based products like yogurt are excellent sources of calcium. Calcium absorption is also aided by acidity in the digestive tract. Too much fat, *oxalic acid* (found in spinach, rhubarb, and chocolate), and *phytic acid* (found in grains) in the diet can result in calcium not being absorbed. The recommended calcium-phosphorous ratio is one-to-one, but this is almost impossible to achieve, especially in diets as high in protein as that of the average American. In general, meats, poultry and fish supply fifteen to twenty times more phosphorous than calcium, whereas eggs, grains, nuts, dried beans, and lentils provide about twice as much phosphorous. Data from studies suggest that high phosphorous intakes

CALCIUM SOURCES

VERY GOOD	GOOD
Milk, especially skim and low-fat yogurt	Potatoes
Cheese	Oranges
Sardines	Figs
Kidney beans	Oysters
Almonds	Sunflower seeds
Beet greens	Kelp
Broccoli	Soybeans
Salmon	Tofu
Kale	
Watercress	
Bok choy	

or low calcium-to-phosphorous ratios cause bone demineralization and soft tissue calcification. Evidence indicates that both protein and phosphorous affect the calcium requirement in humans. Calcium retention is believed to be reduced by increases in protein, which intensifies the loss of calcium in urine.[49]

Calcium ingestion may have an effect on mood. Kaymar Arasteh, Ph.D., of Texas A & M University discussed his calcium-mood research at an August 1987 meeting of the American Psychological Association in New York.[50] He reported that depressed patients given 1,000 milligrams of *calcium gluconate* plus 600 international units of vitamin D twice a day for four weeks showed a significant elevation in mood compared to a control group of depressed patients who received placebos. Dr. Arasteh noted that calcium's effect on nerves in the brain and on mood is biphasic—that is, a little stimulates the nerves and elevates mood, but a lot can depress nerve activity and mood.

The RDA's for calcium are 800 to 1,200 milligrams for adults and 360 to 1,200 milligrams for infants and children, but because of the interrelationships among calcium, protein, and phosphorous, many researchers believe it is almost impossible to select a single requirement for any age group.[51] Surveys have shown that American women consume approximately 450 to 550 milligrams of calcium a day, only about half of the amount believed to be needed to help slow age-related bone loss. On the other hand, too much calcium can cause kidney failure, intestinal sluggishness, and psychosis.[52]

Chromium. Chromium allows insulin to regulate blood sugar, which is of vital importance to your brain (see chapter 4). It is believed that a marginal chromium deficiency exists in a large percentage of the population. However, knowledge of chromium absorption and availability is incomplete. Three scientifically sound studies have reported that the elderly and even younger adults may have low levels of chromium and that supplemental chromium seems to have a beneficial effect on carbohydrate tolerance and cholesterol levels. Therefore, some researchers believe that chromium deficiency may play a part in diabetes and arterial disease. Since chromium and insulin work hand in hand, this is not improbable; however, not enough is known about the mineral to set an RDA.[53]

CHROMIUM SOURCES

VERY GOOD	GOOD
Black pepper	Corn oil
Brewer's yeast	Shellfish
Mushrooms	Chicken
Meat products	
Whole grains	

The estimated SDI's for chromium are 0.05 to 0.2 milligrams for adults and 0.1 to 0.08 milligrams for infants and children.

Cobalt. Cobalt, an essential constituent of vitamin B_{12}, was first shown to cause a debilitating, wasting disease in sheep when the amount in the diet was insufficient. Data on the human need for cobalt is sparse and controversial. In research reported by the Russians, cobalt deficiency has been associated with disturbances in thyroid function—and, of course, thyroid hormone is needed for proper brain function.[54] Too much thyroid causes agitation. Too little produces lethargy in adults.[55] Cobalt is most useful when absorbed as part of B_{12}.[56] Vitamin B_{12} is a cobalt-containing compound. Cobalt is also found in green leafy vegetables.

Copper. Copper is a component of several enzymes, including the enzyme needed to make skin, hair, and other pigments. It stimulates iron absorption and is needed to make red blood cells, connective tissue, and nerve fibers. It helps the amino acid tyrosine do its work (tyrosine serves as a raw material for certain brain neurotransmitters). Copper deficiency

COPPER SOURCES

VERY GOOD	GOOD
Almonds	.Beans
Avocados	Dried prunes
Oysters	Walnuts
Margarine	Shrimp
Mushrooms	Bananas
Cocoa	

is rare. Women who use birth control pills have an elevated level of copper in their blood, but the significance of this is unclear.

The estimated SDI's for copper are 2 to 3 milligrams for adults and 0.5 to 1.5 milligrams for infants and children.

Iodine. Two-thirds of the body's iodine is in the thyroid gland, located in the neck. Since the thyroid controls metabolism, and iodine influences the thyroid, an iodine deficiency can result in cloudy thinking, depressed mood, weight gain, and lack of energy in adults. In newborns, cretinism (stunted growth, swollen features, and mental deficiency) occurs with iodine deficiency (see pages 164). A long-term iodine deficiency in adults can result in goiter, the extreme enlargement of the thyroid gland. Foods with *goitrogens* that can block the thyroid's uptake of iodine include cabbage, broccoli, brussels sprouts, kale, turnips, rutabagas, cauliflower, mustard seed and horseradish. Fortunately, because of iodized salt, goiter is rare today.

The RDA's for iodine are 150 micrograms for adults and 40 to 120 micrograms for infants and children.

IODINE SOURCES	
VERY GOOD	GOOD
Kelp and other seaweed	Onions
Seafood	Vegetables grown in iodine-rich soil

Iron. Iron is essential for making hemoglobin, the red substance in blood that carries oxygen to your brain cells, and for making use of that oxygen when it arrives. Iron is widely distributed in the body, mostly in the blood, with relatively large amounts in the liver, spleen, and bone marrow. Your body loses iron mainly through blood loss. Iron-deficiency anemia occurs when there is an inadequate diet, impaired absorption of iron, blood loss, repeated pregnancy, chronic diarrhea, or a greater need for manufacturing blood. This is why women of childbearing age, pregnant women, and growing children are most likely to suffer from iron-deficiency anemia. Symptoms of deficiency include weakness, fatigue, pale skin, and cold feet. When plant foods containing iron, such asparagus and spinach, are eaten with citrus fruits, tomatoes and peppers, or other foods containing vitamin C, iron absorption is increased. Caffeine decreases the absorption of iron, so iron supplements should certainly not be taken with a cup of coffee or cola.

The RDA's for iron are 18 milligrams for adults and 10 to 15 milligrams for infants and children. The average diet yields only 6 milligrams of iron.

IRON SOURCES

VERY GOOD	GOOD
Blackstrap molasses	Green leafy vegetables
Clams	Nuts
Brewer's yeast	Asparagus
Eggs	Oatmeal
Organ meats	Dried peaches
Oysters	Dates, raisins, and prunes
Prune juice	Tofu
Most beans, especially garbanzo and black	Tomato juice
	Pumpkin seeds

Magnesium. Magnesium conducts nerve impulses and keeps the messages going in the brain. It maintains metabolism, aids normal muscle contraction, including that of the heart muscle, and is necessary for kidney, liver, and other organ functions. It is needed by cells for the creation of genetic material. It helps calcium, vitamin C, phosphorous,

MAGNESIUM SOURCES

VERY GOOD	GOOD
Bran buds	Green leafy vegetables
Tofu	Figs
Spinach	Lemons
Brown rice	Yellow corn
Oatmeal	Apples
Soybeans	Apricots
Avocados	Bananas
Beef	Cashews
Blackstrap molasses	Wheat flakes

sodium, and potassium do their jobs in the body. Magnesium is important to the conversion of blood sugar into energy, and it has a reputation for being an antistress mineral because a magnesium deficiency can cause nervousness, irritability, and depression. It is also reported to be vital to exercise endurance. A deficiency also causes muscle weakness, twitching, cramps, and irregular heartbeats. An overdose of magnesium can cause nervous system disorders and can be fatal to people with kidney disease. Ingesting diuretics and alcohol will deplete the level of magnesium in your body.

The RDA's for magnesium are 350 to 400 milligrams for men, 300 milligrams for women, and 50 to 250 milligrams for infants and children.

Manganese. Manganese is essential to enzymes that extract energy from food and convert proteins into amino acids and neurotransmitters. It is needed for normal tendon and bone structure and for some enzymes important to metabolism, particularly in processing glucose and fatty acids. A manganese deficiency in humans is unknown. Animal studies have shown that manganese turns off neuromuscular transmission of signals. It has been suggested that changes in the manganese concentration in human body fluids may be associated with some neurological disorders.[57]

The estimated SDI's for manganese are 2.5 to 5 milligrams for adults and 0.5 to 3 milligrams for infants and children.

MANGANESE SOURCES	
VERY GOOD	GOOD
Nuts	Tea
Unrefined grains	Vegetables
Legumes	Fruits
Soybeans	Coffee

Molybdenum. A component of several enzymes needed in metabolism, molybdenum helps regulate iron storage. There is no known human deficiency. High levels in the diet, however, have been reported to cause a copper deficiency.[58]

The estimated SDI's for molybdenum are 0.15 to 0.5 milligrams for adults and 0.03 to 0.15 milligrams for infants and children.

MOLYBDENUM SOURCES	
VERY GOOD	GOOD
Legumes	Whole-grain cereal
Milk	
Organ meats	

Phosphorous. Phosphorous is involved in nearly all metabolic reactions in the body. It is necessary for nerve and muscle function and for the transmission of messages in the brain. It works with calcium and vitamin D to build strong bones and teeth. Calcium and phosphorous should be consumed in a ratio of two calcium to one phosphorous but rarely is in the Western diet (see pages 51–52). Antacids destroy phosphorous. A deficiency causes weakness and bone pain. An overdose hinders the body's absorption of calcium.

The RDA's for phosphorous are 800 to 1200 milligrams for adults and 240 to 800 milligrams for infants and children.

PHOSPHOROUS SOURCES	
VERY GOOD	GOOD
Meat	Peas
Nuts	Cereal
Seeds	Cheese
Fish	Apricots
Bran	Cocoa
Most beans, especially pinto and black	Tofu
Cottage cheese	Corn
Milk	Almonds
Yogurt	Broccoli

Selenium. Selenium interacts with vitamin E to serve as part of the body's antioxidant defense system. In the 1980s, interest in selenium in human nutrition has grown and the element has been shown to be an essential nutrient.[59] Knowledge about selenium deficiencies and supplementation is sparse. Several reports have indicated that selenium can reduce the incidence of cancer in animals, but as yet this is unproven in

SELENIUM SOURCES	
VERY GOOD	GOOD
Wheat germ	Onions
Bran	Tomatoes
Tuna	Broccoli
Garlic	
Liver	

humans. The range between benefit and toxicity is very narrow with this mineral.[60] Selenium in very small amounts is essential to life, but it is more toxic than arsenic and mercury and less abundant in the earth's crust than gold.

A provisional RDA of selenium is 50 to 200 micrograms for adults. The amount of selenium in the diet depends on the amount contained in the soil and water.

Zinc. Zinc may help regulate chemical communication between brain cells and could be a clue to the chemical basis of learning. It may also help explain how the brain protects itself from certain forms of injury. Stanford University researcher Dennis Choi, M.D., an assistant professor of neurology, and his colleagues reported in 1987 that zinc affects glutamate receptors in the brain (see pages 153).[61] These researchers believe that zinc could serve as a brake that protects against seizures or nerve cell injury. However, too much zinc, they said, can be toxic to brain cells. Zinc is present in all organs and is key in many body processes. It is vital to the activity of more than one hundred enzymes. Zinc aids wound healing, affects reproduction, and counteracts the harmful effects of cadmium. Low zinc levels have been reported in the brains of epileptics and in men suffering from hardening of the arteries. A deficiency in zinc causes impaired cell growth and repair and a reduced sense of taste, and profoundly affects growth in fetuses and children.

A zinc deficiency is also suspected of playing a part in anorexia (self-starvation) and bulimia (characterized by gorging and purging) (see chapter 11). Alexander G. Schauss, Ph.D., director of the American Institute of Biosocial Research in Tacoma, Washington, says that the initial reduction of food intake in anorexics probably results from social influences, but that during adolescence, there are increased demands for most nutrients and for zinc in particular.[62] According to Dr. Schauss, the further zinc levels decline, the more the zinc-dependent senses of taste and smell reduce the desire for food.

When Dr. Schauss and his colleague, Dr. Derek Bryce-Smith, tested the anorexics, they found a zinc deficiency. They described one thirteen-year-old anorexic girl who weighed only 69.5 pounds. She was given 15 milligrams of zinc three times a day. After two weeks, her mood and appetite improved and she smiled; her weight had increased by 3.3 pounds. After several weeks on zinc, her weight rose to 97 pounds and her mood and appetite were reported normal.

Excessive amounts of zinc, on the other hand, can cause nausea, vomiting, abdominal pain, gastric bleeding, premature labor, and still-birth. Zinc megadoses also inhibit calcium absorption if dietary calcium is already low. Similarly, large amounts of iron in the diet can reduce the absorption of zinc. When zinc is present in the diet in adequate amounts, the body makes better use of vitamin A. A lack of zinc can cause night blindness indirectly, by not helping vitamin A to be released from liver stores, even when the diet is sufficient in vitamin A.

The RDA's for zinc are 15 milligrams for adults and 3 to 10 milligrams for infants and children.

ZINC SOURCES

VERY GOOD	GOOD
Oysters	Clams
Whole-wheat bread	Cranberry juice
Wheat bran and wheat germ	Tuna
Beef	Applesauce
Lamb	Cocoa powder
Liver	Peanut butter
Herring	Rice cereal
Most beans, especially black-eyed peas, garbanzos, lentils, and green peas	Eggs
Brown rice	Cooked spinach
Oatmeal	
Soy products	

SUMMING IT UP

There are dietary factors that can affect the absorption and utilization of both vitamins and minerals. It may surprise you to know that fiber—that much-touted anticancer ingredient—and other plant material may interfere. Fiber, phytates, oxalates, and tannins found in plants can attach themselves to certain nutrients and render then them incapable of absorbing through the intestinal wall. The nutrients most commonly affected are calcium, iron, zinc, copper, magnesium, protein, and vitamin B_6.

Fibers, such as bran, that provide bulk in the diet interfere with nutrient availability. Phytates—substances in whole grains, beans, and nuts that bind with zinc, calcium, magnesium, and iron to form a compound the body can't absorb—may lower the levels of these metals, so going overboard and loading yourself with fiber is not a good idea.

Oxalates, which are abundant in spinach, rhubarb, beef, collard greens, soybean products, wheat germ, and Swiss chard, deplete foods of their calcium, even those that are naturally high in calcium, because they keep the calcium from being absorbed. Almonds, cashews, chocolate, and cocoa also contain oxalates.

Tannin and other phenols found in tea and red wine can reduce the availability of iron, vitamin B_{12}, and protein by forming chemical complexes with the enzymes needed to metabolize these nutrients.

Aging, about which we can do little, of course, causes the reduced secretion of stomach acid, which can affect absorption of many important nutrients. Protein, iron, zinc, calcium, and vitamins A, E, folic acid, and B_{12} are among the nutrients possibly affected.

Alcohol and tobacco, as mentioned earlier, generally deplete the body of vitamins. In fact, alcohol interferes with the absorption of all nutrients. You must age, but if you also smoke and drink, dietary supplementation is advisable as an antidote to the effects of abuse. Dietary supplementation may assist the body in other ways in its handling of abuse of these popular drugs and the malabsorption and poor utilization that may occur with aging. Younger people under the stress of striving for athletic or career achievements also may need supplementation. In fact, we may all need vitamin and mineral supplementation, but, as Dr. Baker cautions, "Too much of a good thing is always bad."[63]

So, if you want your brain and body to work well, here are some pointers:

Buy wisely. Some foods have more nutrients than others. Whole-grain cereals and breads are better than refined ones because some of the nutrients are lost during milling and are not restored by "enrichment." Fresh or frozen fruits and vegetables are preferable to canned ones which have been exposed to vitamin-destroying high temperatures. If you do find canned vegetables and fruits more convenient, don't throw out the liquid. Use it in casseroles or soups, because these liquids contain the water-soluble B and C vitamins.

For keep sake. Store frozen foods at zero degrees Fahrenheit or below, and try to use the products within two months. Keep canned foods at about sixty-five degrees and refrigerate greens promptly. Keep milk and bread in opaque containers, as strong light destroys riboflavin. Try to use freshly squeezed oranges or, if you buy cartons of juice, use it as soon as possible. Even overnight storage can deplete orange juice of some of its vitamin C.

Cook right. If you can find your grandmother's old iron cooking pots, you can add this mineral to your meals without cost. To retain water-soluble vitamins, avoid soaking fresh vegetables. Vitamin C can be preserved by preparing salads and vegetables just before serving and by boiling or baking potatoes in the skin. Boil or steam vegetables until just tender, using the least amount of water possible. Pressure-cooking preserves the most vitamins; steaming is second-best. Broiling, frying, or roasting meats preserves more B vitamins than does braising or stewing, unless the broth is also consumed.

One potato two. The white potato, like the banana, is loaded with nutrition. In addition to fiber, it contains B vitamins, vitamin C, potassium, iron, copper, magnesium, phosphorous, iodine, and zinc. The sweet potato has all the above as well as a lot of vitamin A. Eat the peel as well as the inside, because the peel not only seals in the nutrients during cooking, it also contains most of the potato's vitamins and minerals.

Have your vitamin levels checked. If you recognize any of the symptoms of deficiency mentioned in this chapter, ask your physician to take a sample of your blood for testing at a laboratory approved for testing vitamin and mineral levels. You may need some supplementation.

Avoid megadoses of vitamins and minerals. In large doses, vitamins are pharmaceuticals. Without medical supervision, loading yourself with one or more vitamins is unwise.

Eat a varied diet. Avoid eating the same thing day after day, and forgo those fad diets that emphasize one food over all others. A well-balanced, varied diet is the best insurance for your brain and body.

⊲ 4 ⊳

Blood, Brain, and Sugar—
How Carbohydrates Affect You

R IGHT BEFORE *her monthly period and sometimes when she was
depressed, Mary, a thirty-two-year-old schoolteacher, craved
sweets. At such times, she could drink three ice-cream sodas at one
sitting or down a whole box of chocolates. For the rest of the month, she
was able to maintain a well-balanced diet.*

*Jack, a twenty-six-year-old college dropout, had a menial job, despite
a high IQ. He was handicapped by periodic panic attacks and obsessive
thoughts. He constantly wanted to clean things—sterilize them—which
was good for his job but bad for his family and social life.*

*Tommy, age five, was hyperactive in private school and under threat of
expulsion, while his father, an advertising executive, seemingly had the
opposite problem. About an hour after the traditional business lunch,
Tommy's father would fall asleep during creative sessions at the agency.*

All of the above cases histories,* gleaned from medical reports, concern carbohydrate metabolism and the brain.

The effects of carbohydrates on behavior is one of the greatest areas
of medical interest today, but it is an arena of conflict. For every report
of experimental results testing carbohydrates and behavior, a spear is
thrown by another expert criticizing the methods used and killing the
conclusions.

No scientist, of course, would deny that sugar and starches have an

---

*The individuals' identities have been changed.

effect on your brain. The debate is over how much effect they have and over what is normal and what is not. Some researchers feel that of all the foods we eat, sugar has the greatest effect on the brain. They base their opinion on the fact that the carbohydrates you eat are broken down into simple sugars and then converted into glucose by your body. Your other tissues can burn fats and protein as well as carbohydrates, but your brain and nerves can use only glucose as fuel. In fact, the adult human brain uses 180 grams of glucose per day.

All carbohydrates that can be metabolized in humans can easily be converted into glucose. Amino acids from proteins and glycerol from fats stored in the body can also be converted by the cells to glucose if there is a need under certain conditions, such as vigorous exercise or lack of food. Making glucose from fats or proteins, however, is slower and more complex than making it from carbohydrates.

Carbohydrates come in many different shapes and forms, which will be described on pages 65–69, but first you should understand how carbohydrates are used and stored by the body.

Carbohydrates are starches and sugars. Foods rich in carbohydrates are grains, seeds, beans, vegetables, and fruits. Unrefined or complex carbohydrates (nonprocessed) are made up of a long chain of molecules strung together like beads. During digestion, they slowly break down into smaller molecules of glucose. Refined (processed) carbohydrates such as sucrose (table sugar) are made up of short chains of molecules that break down into glucose much faster during digestion. It takes about five minutes for sucrose to begin raising blood-sugar levels. The rapid absorption of sucrose into the blood stream causes a sudden spurt of insulin that, in turn, may cause the blood sugar to fall too fast. Complex carbohydrates, on the other hand, are metabolized more slowly and do not cause the same quick rise and fall in insulin and blood sugar.

The amount of glucose in your blood is largely controlled by your brain, your liver, your pancreas, and your thyroid, adrenal, and pituitary glands. If your blood-sugar level falls too low, your brain sends out an order to your pituitary and thyroid glands to signal your liver to start turning the glycogen from fat in storage into glucose.

Since your brain can't store glucose, it is totally dependent on the glucose it receives from your blood stream. When the glucose level in your blood is low, your brain may not receive enough energy and, therefore, you are unable to think clearly. In extreme cases, when the blood sugar drops too low, the equipment may break down all together and coma and death may result.

Too much sugar in the blood is known as hyperglycemia. Diabetics suffer from this. Too little sugar in the blood is known as hypoglycemia. Victims of low blood sugar suffer from this (see page 70).

Are there certain forms of sugar that are better for your brain than others? That question is under debate. The common sugars are described in the following pages.

Sucrose. White sugar, powdered sugar, brown sugar, maple sugar, beet sugar, turbinado sugar, and raw sugar are all varieties of sucrose. The process used to refine sugar consists of pressing of boiling sliced beets or shredded sugar cane to extract a liquid sugar which is then purified in a series of steps including straining, heating, evaporation, boiling, centrifugation, dissolving, clarification (removal of suspended matter), filtration, crystallization, and drying.

As raw sugar is refined, its molasses content is rinsed away. The remaining sugar is dissolved in warm water to make a syrup, which is filtered repeatedly to remove impurities and color. During this stage, the sugar is referred to as brown sugar, because it retains varying amounts of molasses, depending on the number of filtrations it has undergone. Thus, brown sugar varies in color from very dark brown to light brown. The flavor varies with the color: the lighter the color, the milder the flavor.

The mineral content of brown sugar is greater than that of the more refined product, white sugar. For example, 100 grams of brown sugar (about one-half cup) provides about 3.4 milligrams of iron as compared to the 0.1 milligrams in white sugar, and 385 calories as compared to 373 calories in white sugar.[1] So you get a slight bonus of nutrients and taste from brown sugar. A tablespoon of granulated sugar has 46 calories and 11 grams of carbohydrates. The same amount of powdered sugar has 30 calories and 8 grams of carbohydrates, while brown sugar has 50 calories and 13 grams of carbohydrates. It takes sucrose about five minutes to begin raising blood sugar.[2]

Molasses. Molasses is concentrated syrup from sugar-bearing plants, primarily sugar cane and sugar beets. It is a mixture of sucrose and other materials such as fat and protein and a small amount of minerals such as iron. One tablespoon of molasses has 50 calories and 13 grams of carbohydrates.

Glucose. A sugar that exists naturally in the blood and in grape and corn sugars, glucose is sweeter than sucrose. It is a source of energy for plants and animals. Glucose syrup is used to flavor sausage, hamburger, meat loaf, luncheon meat, and chopped or pressed ham. It is also used as an extender in maple syrup. Five glucose units strung together in long sugar chains form the starch found in wheat, corn, potatoes, and rice. Glucose is two-thirds as sweet as sucrose. It takes two minutes for glucose to start raising blood sugar because no digestion is required. It moves directly through the stomach and intestinal walls into the blood stream.[3]

Fructose, levulose, or fruit sugar. Most fruits contain fructose. The claim that fructose is "natural" appears to be based on the fact that fructose is found naturally in fresh fruit. Table sugar is also natural, however, as it comes from cane sugar. Fresh fruit contains only 20 to 40 percent fructose; the rest of its sugar content is largely sucrose and glucose. Fructose can be up to twice as sweet as sucrose. It is used as a medicine, as a preservative, as a common sugar, and to prevent grittiness in ice cream.

Fructose and sucrose also differ in their ability to stimulate insulin secretion. Sucrose causes the pancreas to secrete a more immediate and probably larger spurt of insulin than does fructose. Scientists think that more insulin is needed to metabolize sucrose because the glucose half of the sucrose requires insulin to be absorbed into the cells or metabolized by the liver. Fructose requires no insulin for the initial stage of metabolism by the liver, but it does require insulin for the portion that is converted to glucose. Thus, fructose does stimulate insulin secretion, but not as rapidly and probably not as much as does glucose. Fructose therefore causes less of a rise and fall in blood-sugar levels than sucrose. Fructose was used in the treatment of diabetes before the introduction of insulin therapy. It is still widely used in Europe in the diabetic diet.[4]

Fructose is about 70 percent sweeter than sucrose, so less is needed as a sweetener in recipes. There are about 48 calories in a tablespoon of fructose and 12 grams of carbohydrate. It takes fructose about twenty-five minutes to start raising your blood-sugar level.[5]

High-fructose corn syrups. Increasingly popular as a sweetener in foods, high-fructose corn syrups are composed of a fifty-fifty mixture of fructose and glucose. It is made by either chemically splitting sucrose into its two component sugars and then separating out and purifying the fructose, or by treating corn syrup with enzymes to convert some of its glucose to fructose. High-fructose corn syrup contains anywhere from 10 to 58 percent glucose. One tablespoon of it has about 58 calories.

Lactose. Also known as milk sugar, saccharum lactin, and D-lactose, lactose is a slightly sweet-tasting, colorless sugar composed of glucose and galactose. *Galactose* is called "brain sugar" because it is found in the covering of the nerves in the brain. Lactose is present in the milk of mammals—humans have 6.7 percent and cows 4.3 percent. It appears commercially as a white powder or crystalline mass, a by product of the cheese industry. Lactose is inexpensive and is widely used in the food industry as a culture medium, such as in souring milk, to maintain moisture, and as a nutrient in formulas for infants and debilitated patients. It is also used as a medical diuretic and a laxative. A number of people are intolerant of lactose, particularly as they grow older. Lactose intolerance results when the enzyme *lactase* is not secreted in sufficient quantities to digest the lactose that has been consumed. The result can be abdominal distention, cramps, and other digestive problems. Lactose has about 50 calories per fluid ounce.

Maltose. Comprised of two glucose units, maltose is found in starch and glycogen. Commercially, its colorless crystals derive from the action of enzymes of the malt extracted from barley on starch. It is soluble in water and is used as a nutrient, as a sweetener, and as a table-sugar substitute for diabetics. It is also used in making beer, maple syrup, and corn syrups and is an ingredient in bread and infant foods. Maltose is only one-third as sweet as sugar or about 126 calories per half cup.

Honey. Honey is a mixture of glucose, fructose, and water. Commonly thought of as pure fructose, honey actually contains as much glucose as fructose. Because of its taste and texture, some people feel that a smaller amount of honey satisfies the desire for sweetness better than table sugar, although there is no real nutritive advantage. Honey has about 65 calories per tablespoon.

Corn syrup. Also known as corn sugar or dextrose, corn syrup is the most common form of dextrose. It consists primarily of glucose (see page 66). Corn syrup is made by heating corn starch, using acids or enzymes as catalysts. It is used in maple, nut, and root-beer flavorings for beverages; ice cream; ices; candies; and baked goods. Corn syrup is also used on envelopes, stamps, and sticker tapes; in ale, aspirin, bacon, baking mixes, powders, beer, bourbon, breads, breakfast cereals, pastries, candy, carbonated beverages, catsup, cheeses, cereals, chop suey, chow mein, confectioners' sugar, cream puffs, fish products, ginger ale, ham, jellies, processed meats, peanut butter, canned peas, plastic food wraps, sherbet, whiskey, and American wines. It is a common allergen. A tablespoon of corn syrup contains about 58 calories and 14.5 carbohydrates.

Starch. Starch is stored by plants and is taken from grains of wheat, potatoes, rice, corn, beans, and many other vegetable foods. Such foods are also rich in fiber and various other nutrients. In many foods, however, the starch is not digestible until it is cooked or processed in some other way. Starches vary in calorie content, but corn starch has about 40 calories and 33 grams of carbohydrates per tablespoon. Starch takes about ten minutes to begin raising blood-sugar levels.[6]

Modified starch. Modified starch is ordinary starch that has been altered chemically to modify such properties as thickening or jelling. Babies have difficulty digesting starch in its original form. Modified starch is used in baby food on the theory that it is easier to digest. Questions about safety have arisen because babies do not have the resistance that adults do to chemicals. Among the chemicals used to modify starch are propylene oxide, aluminum sulfate, and sodium hydroxide (lye).[7]

Since some starches are more digestible and since some sugars are more easily converted to glucose, are some carbohydrates better for your brain than others? As already pointed out, your brain's major fuel is glucose.

Results of studies have raised questions about the blood glucose effects of various carbohydrate sources. There are indications that foods with exactly the same carbohydrate content may have dramatically different effects on blood sugar.[8]

John Bantle, M.D., of the University of Minnesota investigated the effects of different forms of sugar on the glucose levels in the blood of both normal and diabetic subjects.[9] He and his colleagues studied responses to five meals, each containing a different form of carbohydrate but all with nearly identical amounts of total carbohydrate, protein, and fat. The subjects were ten healthy persons, twelve patients with Type I diabetes (requiring insulin injections), and ten patients with Type II diabetes (adult onset, requiring no insulin). The test carbohydrates were glucose, fructose, sucrose, potato starch, and wheat starch. In all three groups, the meal containing sucrose as the test carbohydrate did not produce significantly greater glucose peaks in the blood than did meals containing potato, wheat, or glucose as test carbohydrates. The meal with fructose as the test carbohydrate produced the smallest increments in blood-sugar levels.[10] Dr. Bantle concluded that fructose produces less post-meal blood sugar than do other common types of carbohydrate. But he cautioned that additional research is needed because the long-term effects of substantial amounts of fructose in the diet remain unknown.

Until the mystery is solved, it makes sense to get your sugar as fructose from fruits, vegetables, and other items in which it is a natural part of the product. Like sucrose, fructose contains no real nutritive value; however, it may be more effective than other forms of sugar in suppressing hunger. Since fructose does not cause the dip in blood sugar about two hours after its is eaten that sucrose does, it is not likely to cause the hunger sensation that occurs with the sucrose-caused blood-sugar drop. Therefore, symptoms also associated with low blood sugar—lethargy and/or irritability—may not be as likely to occur when fructose is substituted for sucrose. This, of course, has not been proven. The effects of extreme variations of blood-sugar levels on the brain are well known and accepted. The more subtle effects on the brain of sugar in the diet is the subject of many a debate.

In 1976 and again in 1986, the Federation of American Societies for Experimental Biology evaluated the health effects of sucrose as a food ingredient, and in a report to the FDA stated:

> The panel still believes that sugar consumption has nothing to do with developing diabetes . . . sugar does not affect the level of proteins or fats normally circulating in the blood stream. . . . [I]t isn't the cause of diabetes, and there is no substantial evidence that the consumption of sugar is responsible for behavioral changes in children or adults with the exception of relatively rare hypoglycemias [low blood sugar] in that population.[11]

Alexander Schauss, Ph.D., editor-in-chief of the *International Journal of Biosocial Research,* said in an editorial concerning the federation's report to the FDA that while there may be no definitive cause-and-effect relationships between sugar and behavior, there is some evidence that sugar has adverse effects on all of the health conditions mentioned in the federation's report. "Demanding that researchers demonstrate a clear relationship between sugar intake and medical and behavioral disorders is unrealistic. It reeks of the same tactic used for over 200 years by the tobacco industry," stated Dr. Schauss.[12]

No one argues about the fact that directly after a meal, your glucose level rises. Then, insulin is secreted by your pancreas to help move sugar into your cells, and your glucose level drops. If your blood sugar falls to lower than normal levels following a meal, your brain will send out distress signals. You may feel dizzy, fatigued, weak, and nervous, and your heart may pound—symptoms not unlike those of an acute anxiety attack. However, they are a result not of the low blood sugar, but of too much of the hormone epinephrine (adrenaline), which is sent to signal your liver to make more glucose. There are many debates about whether the afore-mentioned symptoms such as dizziness and fatigue are due to anxiety or to the ingestion of too much refined sugar.

HYPOGLYCEMIA—LOW BLOOD SUGAR

The level of sugar in your blood can vary from 50 to 110 milligrams per deciliter of blood if you are perfectly healthy. A blood-sugar level below 40 milligrams per deciliter is considered hypoglycemic. It is a condition that can be caused by several factors.

Many physicians say that true hypoglycemia is rare and that the diagnosis of "low blood sugar" is often given just because it is more acceptable than attributing symptoms to emotions. But can anxiety cause a drop in blood sugar? And can a drop in blood sugar cause anxiety in a healthy person?

If you do not eat during the night, your body will normally release glucose from your liver stores. Even if you have been starving for days and your liver supply of glucose is exhausted, your body will sacrifice other organs to keep your brain supplied with blood sugar. However, in people with certain diseases (insulin-producing tumors, liver disease, alcoholism, and so forth) and in some with no discernible physical explanation, the blood sugar will gradually drop to abnormally low levels during fasting. Besides the symptoms mentioned earlier, headaches, an inability to concentrate, forgetfulness, and sleepiness will result. This state is known as *fasting hypoglycemia,* a condition that requires a careful search for its underlying cause.

Postprandial (after a meal) hypoglycemia, or *reactive hypoglycemia,* is the most common type. It occurs about two to four hours after eating. A very rapid absorption of glucose into the circulation and a subsequent outpouring of excess insulin causes symptoms such as dizziness, fatigue, weakness, nervousness, and heart palpitations.

The standard test for diagnosing hypoglycemia is the glucose-tolerance test. After an overnight fast, you are given a drink containing a highly concentrated sugar solution. Over the next three to five hours, blood sugars are measured periodically. After drinking the sugar, your blood-glucose level will increase and then drop gradually to normal. But if you are hypoglycemic, your blood sugar will drop sharply several hours after the test and, at the same time, you will develop symptoms such as trembling and irritability. Since the oral glucose test is often stopped after three hours, the period of continued decline is often missed.[13]

Many doctors believe that the glucose tolerance tests are not really accurate. Dan Foster, M.D., professor of internal medicine at the University of Texas Health Science Center in Dallas and editor of *Diabetes,* says he doesn't use the test to diagnose hypoglycemia because he believes that low blood-sugar levels can develop in normal people following this test. Even after ordinary meals, 24 percent of normal people developed blood sugar levels lower than 50 milligrams per deciliter of blood, according to one study.[14] This is why many doctors advise those who suspect they have low blood sugar to have a measurement of blood sugar taken at the time when they experience symptoms or two hours after eating a normal meal.

Another reason the glucose-tolerance test may not identify all those with an abnormal sugar metabolism is that insulin alone is not the only blood-sugar regulator. A newly recognized hormone may play a part in blood-sugar swings that is not evident in the traditional glucose-tolerance test.

In a major contribution to scientific understanding of carbohydrate metabolism, National Institute of Aging (NIA) investigators, in collaboration with University of British Columbia scientists, found that a hormone produced in the gut, *gastric inhibitory polypeptide* (GIP), may be critical for maintaining normal blood-sugar levels.[15]

Because of the higher incidence of diabetes among the elderly, the NIA's Gerontology Research Center Clinical Physiology branch has been studying the phenomenon of declining glucose tolerance with age. A key issue is the degree to which tests of glucose tolerance can predict diabetes, a disease that involves blood vessel deterioration. As many as 50 percent—and some say 70 to 80 percent—of persons over the age of sixty show signs of impaired glucose metabolism.

Normally, the pancreas releases sufficient insulin to clear the blood of excess glucose within two hours. If the blood sugar is too high for the pancreas to clear, GIP comes into play. Hence, if you eat a meal containing a lot of sugar, you activate both insulin and GIP.

The NIA investigators also identified an unusual group of individuals whom they have labeled "disparate performers." These people cannot metabolize glucose given by vein, but they are normal performers on the oral test. They have been shown to overproduce GIP and thus to compensate for the primary trigger, glucose.[16]

GIP's part in providing blood sugar for the brain is not yet known, but what is certain is that insulin does have a profound effect on your brain and behavior. If you doubt the effect of insulin on your brain, consider that diabetics, in whom insulin is absent or inefficient, may become comatose if not supplied with an outside source of the hormone to process their blood sugar. And if you don't believe blood sugar affects mood, remember that "insulin shock" was once used to treat depression. When given a dose of insulin, the patient's blood-sugar level would fall rapidly and a comalike state would occur. Then the patient was given glucose to wake up. After awakening, many of the symptoms of depression and even schizophrenia were relieved.

Insulin shock is an exaggeration of the natural interaction between insulin, glucose, and the brain. Your intestines, liver, and endocrine glands constantly cooperate to ensure that your blood-sugar levels stay within a normal range. When you challenge these systems, either by excessive carbohydrate ingestion or by fasting, your organs' reactions to the challenge can be measured. If your blood-sugar level goes too high after carbohydrate ingestion, that's *hyper*glycemia. The most common cause of hyperglycemia is diabetes. If your blood-sugar level drops too low after carbohydrate ingestion, that's *hypo*glycemia.

Because the glucose-tolerance test does not identify some people who do react adversely to refined sugar, Dr. Larry Christensen, of Texas A & M University, and his colleagues sought to develop a test that could identify these individuals. At the August 1987 meeting of the American Psychological Association, Dr. Christensen pointed out:

> Although most of the evidence has focused on the impact of carbohydrates in general as opposed to refined sucrose, we have, in our laboratory, obtained data suggesting that refined sucrose ingestion can produce symptoms such as depression, confusion, and fatigue in selected individuals.[17]

He emphasized *selected* individuals, since some people are unaffected.

Dr. Christensen and his group studied a group of volunteers who answered newspaper ads calling for persons with the following symptoms: "depressed, tired, feeling bad most of the time."

After two series of studies, the Texas researchers developed the 62-item Christensen Dietary Distress Inventory Scale, which contains cognitive, behavioral, and physiological items that can help identify those who are "dietary-mood responders." Dr. Christensen indicated that the scale still needs to be refined, but that it should help diagnose those patients whose blood-glucose tests are normal but who, indeed, are affected cognitively and emotionally by the ingestion of refined sugar.

Whether or not you are hypersensitive to refined sugar, you can still cause significant changes in your blood-sugar level by what you eat, and such changes can affect your brain function and behavior.

BREAKFAST

Breakfast—its very name says a lot about its effects on your body. The early part of the waking day is a period that is generally associated with the upward phase of the circadian rhythm, when there is a rapid increase in levels of alertness, arousal, and activation. It seems logical that breaking a fast would affect the level of sugar found in the brain and get the central processor revved up. Many of us cannot even communicate with others in our households until we have had our glass of orange juice or cup of coffee after awakening.

Dr. Ernesto Pollitt of the University of Texas had half a group of children skip breakfast while the another half ate a meal of waffles and syrup, milk, and orange juice. By late morning, those who had eaten breakfast made fewer errors solving problems than the children who had skipped breakfast.[18]

These results in short-term incidental memory and problem-solving accuracy were interpreted as being the result of attitude. That is, when the subjects missed breakfast, they were more likely to become fatigued. As a result, they were more excitable, had a harder time concentrating, and were not performing as well as they usually did.[19]

Jason, mentioned at the beginning of this chapter, is a dramatic example of the effect of breakfast on the brain. He was chronically obsessive and, despite his high IQ, couldn't stop thinking about the presence of germs long enough to concentrate on his schoolwork. Neither psychological treatment nor medications had helped him.

A twenty-six-year-old university dropout, Jason had a fifteen-year history of psychotherapy and drug treatment for panic attacks and discomfort. He also suffered from acne, constipation, and hypertension. Hospitalization did not help him overcome his obsession. He reported that his panic attacks preceded a worsening of his obsessions, and that fluctuations in panic attack severity coincided with fluctuations in both his mood and his acne problem. These factors suggested a common, possibly dietary, cause.

Although he was skeptical about the ability of diet to help where so many previous orthodox treatments had failed, Jason was willing to try anything. He felt he had nothing to lose. Jason was put on a hypoallergenic diet that eliminated such foods as cereal, grain, milk, eggs, chicken, chocolate, sugar, caffeine, pork, and chemical additives. He also was given a moderate course of nutritional supplements aimed at preventing obvious deficiencies. After several weeks on the hypoallergenic diet, a high-protein breakfast—consisting of a normal-sized portion of meat, fish, or poultry, with or without a piece of low-carbohydrate fresh fruit— was added.

Jason has remained free of obsessions for twenty-three months. His prompt response to the addition of the high-protein breakfast to his regimen gave his doctors a clue that he might be suffering from reactive hypoglycemia. A two-hour glucose-tolerance test confirmed their suspicions. His blood-glucose level dropped very low after the standard dose of glucose and, at the same time, he began to develop the mental discomfort that set off his former panic attacks.

It was Jason's lack of a high-protein breakfast to regulate his blood-sugar level that caused his problems. Food sensitivity, his doctors believe, contributed to his difficulties, but he was gradually able to reintroduce the eliminated foods, with the exception of alcohol, without bringing back his symptoms.[20]

Tommy, mentioned at the beginning of this chapter, liked highly sugared, artificially colored cold cereals. He also loved the cookies his mother baked and the candy his grandmother gave him every time he visited her. His mother, on the advice of Tommy's pediatrician, gave her son warm oat cereal for breakfast and substituted fruit for cookies in his lunch. He was just as happy with frozen natural juice bars as he had been with candy as a treat. Tommy was not part of a controlled study and his improvement could be attributed to the attention he received from his parents about his food or to the fact that he had matured a little more. Nevertheless, his behavior in school was no longer a problem.

In millions of homes, children like Tommy are sent off to school after eating highly sugared cereals. Research by Betty Li and P.J. Schuhmann of U.S. Department of Agriculture's Nutrient Composition Laboratory analyzed sixty-two ready-to-eat breakfast cereals for their sugar content. They found that only three of the sixty-two cereals apparently had no added sugar, two contained more than 50-percent sugar, and the sugar content of the rest fell between these two levels (see page 178).[21]

Tommy's change in diet—from highly sugared foods to complex carbohydrates—not only made him feel better but also had a beneficial effect on the entire family. Seeing the improvement in his son's behavior, Tommy's father decided to change his own diet. Instead of his heavy, fat-and-sugar-laden lunches, he ate a salad or broiled fish and skipped the traditional cocktail. He found that he had much more energy in the afternoon.

And, of course, the mother and wife in the family had more energy and felt better because she no longer had to contend with her son's and husband's behavior problems.

TIMING OF MEALS

Tommy and his father are good examples of the effect of breakfast and lunch on behavior, although the carbohydrates affected them differently. It seems to have made Tommy more active and his father less active. The paradoxical effects could be due not only to their physiological reactions to carbohydrates but also to the time of day they were ingested.

The focus has been on the effects of carbohydrates on the brain and behavior associated with breakfast and lunch because these two meals are immediately relevant to efficiency during the working day. Particular attention has been paid to lunch because it has long been recognized that lunch produces the most obvious behavioral response to food intake.[22]

Researchers have reported (and most of us have found it to be true) that there is a dip in alertness and efficiency at about 2:00 P.M., one or two hours after lunch. There are no such obvious efficiency changes in the morning after breakfast nor later in the day following the evening meal.

Bonnie Spring, Ph.D., Harris Lieberman, Ph.D., and their colleagues at Texas Tech University, found in their studies that subjects who ate a high-carbohydrate lunch felt less alert than those who ate a high-protein lunch. The Texas group had expected just the opposite. They assumed that a high-carbohydrate breakfast would have more powerful effects than the same food eaten for lunch. The rationale was that at lunchtime, one may still be digesting breakfast and may already have somewhat elevated levels of insulin; thus the effects of lunchtime carbohydrates would be blunted. In contrast, the investigators assumed, insulin levels and plasma-amino levels would be low at breakfast, after having fasted for approximately twelve hours. Thus, the high-carbohydrate meal was expected to have its greatest impact at breakfast. Instead, most of the participants in their studies reported that after lunch, mental slump and feelings of fatigue were greater with a high-carbohydrate meal than with a high-protein one.[23]

In an earlier study, Bonnie Spring, Ph.D., formerly of Harvard University, found that adults had difficulty performing a simple speech test after eating a sherbet-like, high-carbohydrate snack. The decline was especially marked for those over age forty. Her tests also showed differences in the way men and women felt after eating the sherbet: women had a more pronounced reaction and reported feeling lethargic and sleepy, while men simply reported feeling calmer.[24]

The Texas Tech researchers are not sure about the interplay between regular circadian rhythms and the nutrient content of the meals, since it has been shown there are regular patterns of rises and falls in mental functions throughout the day. For example, perceptual search tasks may improve over the day, reaching a maximum at 8:00 P.M., while scores on tests that require short-term memory climb to a maximum at 11:00 A.M.

Angus Craig, Ph.D., of the University of Sussex in Brighton, England, wrote in *Nutrition Reviews* that the observed effects of eating a meal depend on the delay between ingesting the food and taking measurements. Observations made within one or two hours of starting a meal may differ considerably from those obtained after three hours. The effects also depend on the gap in time since the previous meal and on the time of day the test meal is eaten.[25]

Dr. Craig and his colleagues also found a dip in efficiency after lunch was eaten, but no change in performance when no lunch was consumed. This led the Sussex university investigators to conclude that with some exceptions, lunch does have an adverse effect on performance for at least two hours afterward, whereupon the effect starts to wane.

Dr. Craig's group also discovered that accuracy on a simple test involving searching a page of type and crossing out all of the *e*'s was significantly influenced after lunch. The test was influenced both by the size of the test lunch eaten and by the size of the lunch ordinarily consumed. The effects on this "search and perceive" test of a heavy, three-course test meal seemed to be less for the person who normally consumed such a meal than for one who normally ate a light lunch.

There are many debates about the association between high-carbohydrate and high-protein meals, time of day, cognition, and mood. None is more heated than the controversy over whether there is a correlation between high sugar intake and hyperactive behavior.

SUGAR, ATTENTION DEFICIT, AND HYPERACTIVITY

The belief that sugar causes behavior and learning problems in children is widely held by the general public and has the support of some noted health professionals. Behavior and learning problems following sucrose consumption have been attributed to a drop in blood sugar or allergic reactions.

Some research studies have concluded that sugar does adversely affect children's behavior and ability to learn, while others have said there is no correlation.

In one recent study, Ronald Prinz, Ph.D., an associate professor of clinical psychology, and David Riddle, a doctoral candidate, under a grant from the National Institute of Child Health and Human Development, found a correlation between sucrose consumption and observed behavior in hyperactive and nonhyperactive four- to seven-year-old children. Mothers kept seven-day food records of the children's intake. At the end of the week, each child was videotaped while playing in a playroom. The trained observers who scored the videotapes were completely unaware of the children's characteristics and dietary intakes, and in fact were not even informed that dietary data had been collected. The observers were highly accurate in estimating the hyperactive group's estimated sucrose consumption. Dr. Prinz concluded that there "may be an association between diets characterized by a high sucrose component and reduced attentional performance in normal boys."[26]

In another recent experiment, further evidence was added that hyperactive children may be more susceptible than others to the effects of sugar on behavior. C. Keith Conners, Ph.D., and his colleagues at the George Washington University School of Medicine and the Children's Hospital National Medical Center reported at the August 1987 meeting of the American Psychological Association on the difference in reactions to sucrose between hyperactive and normal children.[27]

Hyperactive and normal children were assigned to receive one of three breakfasts—high carbohydrate, high protein, or fasting. On two separate days, each group received an aspartame challenge or a sucrose challenge at breakfast. Prior to eating breakfast, blood was withdrawn from a forearm vein by an indwelling catheter that was maintained throughout the testing day. Subsequent samples were drawn at 30, 60, 90, 120, 180 and 240 minutes. Samples were assayed for blood sugar, insulin, growth hormones, cortisol, lactate, glucagon, and fatty acids.

The children sat in a booth and performed a continuous task. This task was repeated in mid- and late morning. Errors of omission, commission, and reaction time were recorded.

Results showed the same pattern of results across performance and hormonal measures. In each case, there was a difference between the hyperactive and normal children who had eaten the high-carbohydrate breakfast but not with the high-protein or fasting breakfast. Errors of omission were significantly worse for hyperactives when sugar was added to the high-carbohydrate breakfast but not when added to the high-protein or fasting breakfast.

Dr. Conners and his group believe the effect of the sugar-carbohydrate diet on behavioral changes was due to the increase in serotonin the combination caused. The researchers propose that either hyperactive children are more sensitive to a rise in serotonin or serotonin interferes with the regulation of dopamine and norepinephrine in the brain. "Sugar may not be harmful to normals but may interfere with cognitive function in hyperactives when they have a carbohydrate load prior to sugar ingestion," Dr. Conners concluded.[28]

Judith Rapoport, M.D., chief of the Child Psychiatry branch of the National Institute of Mental Health, conducted a study of children she described as "sugar responders." Twenty-one children were given behavioral tests after ingesting glucose, sucrose, saccharin, or a placebo. Dr. Rapoport concluded that the children were less active after having ingested the sugar than before, and that "it doesn't seem likely that any of these substances produce significant effects, even in a group of presumed 'sugar reponders.' "[29]

The effect of sugar on behavior is of great interest not only to parents and teachers but also to penal authorities. Studies in prisons are just as controversial as the studies in schools. Here are a few of the studies on sugar and the behavior of offenders:

• In 1971, Barbara Reed, an Ohio probation officer, advocated dietary reform for all of her probationers. She had found that when she eliminated sugary junk foods, white flour, and canned foods from her diet, she felt much better. She reported that clients who followed her dietary instructions also reported feeling better, more energetic, and more emotionally stable. But what really intrigued other law-enforcement agencies was that the rate of recidivism among her charges plunged.[30]

• Stephen Schoenthaler, Ph.D., director of the Social Justice Program at California State College at Stanislaus, began a study of juveniles at the Tidewater Detention Center in Chesapeake, Virginia, in 1980 to see if there was a correlation between sugar and antisocial behavior.[31] He restricted white sugar and substituted fruit juice for colas and honey for table sugar. Whole-wheat breads replaced white bread and brown rice replaced white rice. Processed foods were replaced with fresh produce (when available) and high-sugar, high-fat foods were replaced with more nutritious items. For example, potato chips, ice cream, and cookies were replaced with fresh fruit, fresh vegetables, and a variety of nuts and cheeses. In the study, there was a 48-percent decline overall in antisocial behavior. For the year following the change in diet policy, violence declined by 33 percent, theft dropped 77 percent, insubordination fell 55 percent, horseplay or hyperactivity dropped 65 percent, and rule violations declined by 30 percent.

• Diana Fishbein, a University of Baltimore criminologist, also explored diet and violence and explained why such improvement in behavior as described above may be so spectacular. She pointed out that the brain uses 50 percent of all glucose in the blood. Therefore, when blood-sugar levels are too low, the brain cannot function well and, consequently, behavior is affected. She said that research suggests that low blood sugar may contribute to irritability, headaches, agitation, frustration, and explosive behavior.[32]

Dr. Schoenthaler reasons that chronic deficiencies in elements essential to glucose metabolism, such as zinc, iron, phosphorous, and magnesium, may contribute to the deprivation of chemical energy needed by the brain for intellectual functioning. If there is an energy shortage, the limbic system—the most primitive part of the brain—gets priority because it controls involuntary muscle responses, such as those for breathing and pumping blood as well as those for emotions. The region sacrificed might be that which contributes to reasoning.[33]

A few prison systems have established modified diets for inmates. Their success has not yet been determined. Researchers that have attacked the validity of the studies correlating antisocial behavior and high-sugar diets point out that prison inmates reside in a limited environment that fosters boredom, frustration, and reduced self-esteem. So the presence of researchers in the institution generates interest. Since research projects done in prisons are so noticeable, it is almost impossible to do a controlled study.

CARBOHYDRATE CRAVINGS

Among the unanswered questions about nutrition is why do all of us crave sweets?

The 1986 meeting of the American Psychological Association in Washington, D.C., included a symposium on carbohydrate craving. Dr. Bonnie Spring, who chaired the event, pointed out that carbohydrate craving is a newly recognized symptom that spans several diagnostic categories, positing difficulties for weight management. Said Dr. Spring:

> Recent studies indicate that foods rich in carbohydrate but poor in protein induce drowsiness and impair concentration in healthy adult human subjects. Carbohydrate-rich foods induce greater fatigue and performance impairments than isocaloric [calorie-equal] foods that are high in protein. Yet, some individuals crave and selectively consume large quantities of carbohydrates, raising questions about the causes for this phenomenon. Carbohydrate cravers constitute a substantial subgroup of several clinical populations, including patients with bulima, seasonal affective disorders, obesity and smoking withdrawal. Recent findings suggest that carbohydrate cravers respond differently to carbohydrates than do more balanced eaters. Specifically, carbohydrates may have an antidepressant effect on the mood of individuals who crave them.[34]

Carbohydrate Craving in Obesity   Judith Wurtman, Ph.D., of MIT's food and nutrition department, presented a paper at the same symposium on carbohydrate craving and obesity.[35] She said she and her colleagues identified two groups of obese individuals who consume excessive calories primarily as snack foods: carbohydrate cravers, whose snacks consist mainly of carbohydrate-rich foods, and non-carbohydrate cravers, who consume about equal amounts of carbohydrate- and protein-rich foods as snacks. In a study performed at the MIT Clinical Research Center, they measured mood states before and after the consumption of a carbohydrate-rich lunch by the two classes of obese snackers. After the meal, the moods of the two groups of subjects differed significantly. The non-carbohydrate cravers reported feeling considerably less vigorous, more fatigued, and more sleepy than were the carbohydrate cravers. Moreover, after the high-carbohydrate meal, they rated themselves more depressed, whereas the carbohydrate cravers reported themselves as less depressed. A subgroup of obese individuals, then, may avoid consuming carbohydrate rich-foods by themselves because of the negative effects these foods have on their moods. In contrast, obese carbohydrate cravers may prefer to consume carbohydrate-rich snacks alone because of their positive effects on mood.

In another study, obese carbohydrate cravers were treated with a placebo or with fenfluramine, a drug that enhances the release of serotonin. Fenfluramine significantly reduced carbohydrate snacking.[36]

Conceivably, excessive carbohydrate cravings reflect inadequate serotonin levels in the obese craver's brain, and the craver learns to desire foods that enhance serotonin. For such individuals, carbohydrate intake may be reinforced by an improvement in mood.

Smoking and Carbohydrates Many people are afraid to stop smoking because they fear they will gain weight. And many do—five to ten pounds on the average—but there is no unanimous opinion as to why.

Neil Grunberg, Ph.D., and Deborah Bowen also reported at the 1986 American Psychological Association symposium on carbohydrate cravings that recent human and animal studies indicate that body-weight gains after smoking cessation or after chronic nicotine administration are partially a result of increased consumption of sweet-tasting carbohydrates.[37]

Nicotine affects the availability of glucose. Ex-smokers consume carbohydrates in order to alter the almost unbearable unpleasantness of tobacco abstinence. In effect, carbohydrates might be considered a self-administered tranquilizer. This theory is consistent with reported effects of carbohydrates on mood.

The good news is that most people who continue to eat a regular diet after giving up smoking will gain weight for three months, plateau for two months, and then lose the added weight after five months if they can forego binging on carbohydrates.[38]

SAD-ness and Carbohydrate Craving Another newly recognized, carbohydrate-associated problem, seasonal affective disorder (SAD), was also discussed at the 1986 American Psychological Association meeting. It is a condition in which people become depressed in fall and winter and are fine in the spring and summer. Most SAD victims are women whose symptoms began in their twenties or thirties. In addition to sadness and social withdrawal, these women suffer from overeating, carbohydrate craving, and weight gain.

Norman Rosenthal, M.D., of the National Institute of Mental Health's psychobiology section, was one of the first to identify SAD.[39] He reported that carbohydrate craving occurred in the winter months in 79 percent of SAD patients he and his colleagues studied. Carbohydrate craving is an early symptom, frequently beginning in September or October, generally before mood is affected. Some patients craved sweets and chocolates, whereas others preferred starches. Several patients used terms such as "compulsion," "craving" and "pressure to eat." Like the other symptoms, their cravings almost always subsided in the spring.

Patients who have traveled during the winter months have reported feeling better when they are closer to the equator. Those who moved to more southern locations have reported an overall improvement in their symptoms.

These seasonal changes in mood and behavior resemble the annual rhythms found in a wide variety of animal behaviors, Dr. Rosenthal maintains. So-called circannual rhythms are often synchronized in animals by day length, an effect generally mediated by the nocturnal secretion of melatonin by the pineal gland in the center of the brain. The pineal gland was thought to be the "third eye," and until the 1950s, it was thought to have no real purpose. It is now believed to be a sort of "biological clock" that sends out "ticks" to influence the activities of hormones.

In the thirty-one SAD patients studied by Dr. Rosenthal his associates, winter symptoms, carbohydrate cravings included, were reversed by exposing the patients to light. Symptoms were alleviated with the administration of five to six hours per day of bright, full-spectrum light of an intensity to suppress melatonin. When the patients were then given 2 milligrams per day of melatonin, their depressive symptoms did not recur but their carbohydrate craving became significantly worse. Luncheon meals containing different proportions of carbohydrates and protein were fed to sixteen of the SAD patients. The effects of these meals on mood and performance were evaluated using self-report mood scales and a pencil and paper performance task. For comparison purposes, sixteen normal volunteers matched for sex and mean age were given similar meals. Mood and performance data were analyzed. Plasma amino acid levels were also examined to confirm the experimental manipulation.

According to Dr. Rosenthal, it is conceivable that for patients with SAD, overeating—particularly of carbohydrates—may be part of a complex behavioral feedback loop involving efforts to keep the brain's neurochemicals in balance.

Carbohydrates and the Brains of Bulimics   June Chiodo, Ph.D., of Texas Technical University, in still another paper presented at the 1986 symposium on carbohydrates, linked carbohydrate cravings to bulimic behavior.[40] The intake of high-carbohydrate foods by bulimics is characterized by extremes. Between binges, bulimics typically practice severely restrictive dieting, which may include avoidance of carbohydrates. In contrast, binges are characterized by the rapid intake of large quantities of foods, often involving high-calorie carbohydrates. Binges are usually triggered by feelings of tension, anxiety, or depression. The ingestion of food provides some relief from emotional distress, at least initially. By the end of a binge, however, bulimics report self-deprecating thoughts and typically vow never to binge again. They may also engage in purging behaviors.

The parallels between eating disturbance and emotional disturbance are impressive in bulimics, which suggests they might be interrelated. The first possibility is that dietary restrictions in the interval between binges play a role in perpetuating or exacerbating the affective disturbance. This hypothesis is supported by the evidence that depression increases in proportion to the number of meals skipped and by the finding that brain serotonin-depleting interventions—which include carbohydrate restriction—may induce depression.

The second possible relationship is that carbohydrate-rich dessert-type foods may have an antidepressant effect on bulimics. Data from Dr. Chiodo's laboratory suggest such an effect. It is believed that binging is an unwitting attempt to self-medicate uncomfortable mood states. Since the antidepressant effects of binge eating are short-lived, however, and since they may involve sweet foods that are high in protein as well as carbohydrates, it is doubtful that pharmacologic effects on brain serotonin represents a sufficient explanation mechanism. Dr. Chiodo purports that dessert foods are psychologically reinforcing. In our society, they represent "treats."

SUGAR SENSE

Eat hard fiber. Diets that are high in fiber and carbohydrates are associated with lower blood-glucose and serum-lipid levels. There is no significant difference in the blood sugar response between whole-meal bread and white bread or between white and brown spaghetti. But when white flour is given in the form of spaghetti, blood-glucose levels rise much less than they do when the same amount of white flour is given in the form of bread, which suggests that food form rather than fiber content may be important in determining the blood-sugar response. It has been suggested that the hard form (spaghetti) reduces the starch's accessibility to digestive enzymes.[41]

Eat more raw foods. The way a food is cooked can also result in alterations in the blood-sugar response to a food. Studies have indicated that ingestion of raw starches such as purified amylopectin or corn starch causes a much flatter blood-sugar and insulin response as compared to cooked forms of these starches. Increasing the percentage of raw food in the diet has been suggested in the past as an aid to controlling blood glucose.

Total your carbohydrates each day. The carbohydrates in one meal affect the assimilation of carbohydrates in the next meal. Studies of carbohydrates given in a slowly digested form indicate that they have physical effects not only during and immediately following the time the carbohydrate is ingested but also at the time of subsequent standard meals, where they seem to improve the body's carbohydrate tolerance. Breakfasts containing lentils, which are associated with flattened glycemic and insulin responses, are followed by significantly flatter blood-sugar responses to a standard lunch as compared to breakfasts containing identical amounts of carbohydrate in the form of bread.

Give carbohydrates time to reach your brain. By eating slowly, you can mimic the effects of a slow-release carbohydrate. Thus, bread eaten continuously at an even rate—small portions eaten over four hours— results in a blood-sugar pattern similar to that of a relative portion of lentils eaten within fifteen to twenty minutes. Similar effects are seen when a comparative amount of glucose is sipped slowly over a four-hour period.

Don't drink liquids with your sugary foods. It has been demonstrated that ingestion of a sugar in the liquid part of a meal results in a different metabolic response than when the sugar is ingested in the solid part of a meal. This may be due to the fact that liquids make the contents of your stomach pass through more rapidly; sugar may then be absorbed more quickly into the blood stream through the small intestine.[42]

Time your carbohydrates. Since studies have shown that some people are adversely affected by eating a high-carbohydrate lunch and, conversely, may be positively affected by eating a high-carbohydrate dinner, if you find you are so affected, create and time your meals accordingly.

Exercise if you crave sweets. Gerald Reaven of the Stanford University School of Medicine questions whether we have gone too far on high-carbohydrate diets. The low-fat diets currently in vogue are also high in carbohydrates. Says Reaven, "Anyone who consumes more carbohydrates has to dispose of the load by secreting more insulin."[43] A slim, physically fit person is already very sensitive to insulin and secretes only a small amount in response to carbohydrates. But diabetics and hypertensives secrete much more insulin because their tissues are relatively insensitive to insulin. People with hypertension have higher blood sugar and insulin than people who don't have hypertension.[44]

Don't have sodas and other empty calories in the house. Candy, pastries, sugar-containing soft drinks (some colas have as much as ten teaspoons of sugar in each glass), and alcoholic beverages should be avoided because they cause a rebound drop in blood sugar. If you don't have them at hand, you won't be as tempted and your intake will be cut way down.

Try all-fruit butters and jams. Naturally sweetened fruit butters and jams in place of sugar-sweetened jellies and jams may not reduce your sugar intake by much, but they do have more nutrients than the regular kinds.

Keep fresh fruits handy. Fructose, as we have seen, is more easily metabolized by the body. You will take in a lot of nutrients with it if you opt for fruit.

Eat six to seven small meals per day. If you feel that you may have the symptoms of low-blood sugar described in this chapter, consult your physician. If he or she okays it, try eating small meals more frequently. In that way, you can keep your blood-sugar level more even.

We Westerners do ingest a tremendous amount of refined carbohydrates—about 127 pounds of sugar per person per year, of which 3 percent comes in natural form from fruits and vegetables, 3 percent comes from dairy products, and the balance comes from sugar added to foods. Whether we do it or a food processor does it, sugar added to our food provides an average of 15 to 17 percent of the total calories for adults and 20 to 25 percent for children. The sugar mills worldwide have been working hard to meet the demand. Annual production of sugar has increased from about 18.4 million tons in 1915 to about 97.5 million tons in 1985.[45]

If you use your brain, which uses glucose, you can cut down on refined, highly sugared, empty-calorie foods. You can achieve the following benefits:

1. You'll be less hungry. Robert E. Hodges and W. H. Krehl pointed out in the *American Journal of Clinical Nutrition* that participants in experiments complained of hunger on high-sugar diets but said they felt "stuffed" on sugar-free diets containing complex carbohydrates.[46]

2. Your cholesterol level will drop. A diet high in refined sugars and carbohydrates raises blood cholesterol and other fats, while a diet high in complex carbohydrates lowers blood fats. Research has also established that cholesterol drops if sugar in the diet is replaced with green leafy vegetables, whole grains, and the carbohydrates from legumes.[47]

3. You will avoid wide mood swings and improve your energy level and intellectual ability.

⚔ 5 ⚔

Using Food to Protect Your Brain Against Stroke and Other Damage

---

D o potato chips and other salty foods cause depression, irritability, or stroke?

Can potassium and certain fats protect your brain from damage?

The answer may be yes to all of the above. There is growing evidence that salty foods and certain fats cause damage to brain cells, while potassium and other fats may protect against harm. There is, of course, a great deal of controversy surrounding all of this, even the salt connection, but most agree that diet does play a part. The dispute is over which elements in the diet are significant and to what degree they are significant.

You can certainly affect your brain function by the amount of sodium and potassium you ingest. These two elements in your body fluids are *electrolytes*—dissolved salts or ions—similar to the electrolytes in an automobile battery. Electrolytes "charge" your body and brain with electrical currents and participate in a great variety of chemical processes. These elements are in constant motion within your body. If you are a man, your body is about 55 to 65 percent water, and if you are a woman, about 45 to 55 percent of your body consists of water. About two-thirds of your total body water is within your cells and one-third is between your cells. The level of water in your body is regulated by how thirsty you are, by the antidiuretic hormone released by your pituitary gland, and by your kidneys. In addition to the water you drink, about another 200 to 300 milliliters of water is formed in your body tissues each day. The principal regulator of water and electrolyte balance in your body is your kidneys.

Should your electrolytes become off-balanced, your brain would be the first organ to sound the alert. The warning signals could start with subtle changes in your state of mind. You might feel irritable. If the imbalance develops unchecked, seizures, coma, and death could result.[1]

Many things can upset your electrolyte balance. You can cause occasional imbalances just by being under stress or by jogging too long or not drinking enough fluid in very hot weather. Serious imbalances can result from many other conditions, including vomiting, diarrhea, kidney or liver disease, congestive heart failure, dehydration, severe burns, diabetes, drug treatments, surgery, and edema (water retention), to name a few.

You may not have control over the serious illnesses and accidents that can severely affect your electrolyte balance, but you do have a great deal of control over your diet. Therefore, you can help prevent yourself from falling victim to a number of disabilities involving electrolytes, including stroke and heart disease.

POTASSIUM PROTECTION

Potassium is readily absorbed through the digestive tract; excess amounts are excreted through the kidneys. You need potassium in order to contract your muscles, send messages between your nerves, and release energy from your food. Potassium also dilates blood vessels in the brain and aids circulation. If your potassium level falls, you may feel lethargic and weak. If it falls really low, it can disrupt your heart rhythm and cause kidney and lung failure.

An excess of potassium can result from kidney failure, dehydration, massive injuries, or major infections. Too much potassium can cause nausea, diarrhea, muscle paralysis, and irregular heartbeat. That is why there is a warning on salt-substitute labels. Table salt substitutes may contain 2,700 milligrams of potassium per teaspoon. If potassium were totally substituted for sodium in the American diet, many people would be consuming three times the recommended amount of potassium.

The RDA's for potassium are 1,875 to 5,625 milligrams for adults and 350 to 3,000 milligrams for infants and children.

Despite the recommended intakes and the fact that the adult body contains more than twice as much potassium as sodium, the typical American diet contains less potassium than sodium. A market basket

POTASSIUM SOURCES

VERY GOOD	GOOD
Butternut squash	Yogurt
Bananas	Chicken
Papaya	Dates
Cantaloupe	Salt-free tuna
Raisins	Many salt-substitute foods
Peanuts	Mushrooms
Avocados	Tomatoes
Potatoes	Lima beans
Orange juice	
Brussels sprouts	
Black beans	
Cooked white beans (soy, pinto, and navy)	
Spinach	
Dried apricots	
Skim milk	
Flounder	

survey conducted by the FDA in 1978 indicated that the typical adult consumes nearly 7,000 milligrams of sodium a day and only 4,735 milligrams of potassium.[2] This satisfies the recommendations for potassium, but the distorted balance between potassium and sodium may be a problem for some people.

This imbalance results from the large amounts of sodium added in food processing, in cooking, and at the table. For example, a three-and-a-half-ounce serving of fresh garden peas contains less than one milligram of sodium and 160 milligrams of potassium. Canned peas have 230 milligrams of sodium and 180 milligrams of potassium.

Considerable evidence indicates that the human species evolved on a diet naturally low in sodium and high in potassium. This would explain why the body has such a powerful mechanism for keeping whatever sodium it gets, but readily eliminates potassium. People in developing countries who still live on a high-potassium, low-sodium diet of fruits, nuts, grains, and other plant foods, rarely have high blood pressure.

SALTING YOUR BRAIN

You don't have to be a scientist to recognize that salty foods make you thirsty. That's why peanuts are available at bars. Salt locks a considerable amount of water into your body, and this fluid retention can affect your brain. The symptoms may range from irritability—as victims of premenstrual syndrome know—to unconsciousness and death, as in the case of kidney failure or hydrocephalus (water on the brain). This is the rationale for low-sodium diets, which are designed to ease water-logged tissues of their burden. But a gross deficiency of sodium may produce leg cramps and other types of distress. Correction of electrolyte deficits or excesses is an important part of the management of many ills.

Salty foods not only make you retain fluid, they also raise your blood pressure. More than sixty-million Americans—one in every four—have some form of high blood pressure.[3] Americans have a high sodium intake, about two to two and one-half teaspoons of salt a day. High blood pressure is the most important known risk factor for serious strokes involving the hemorrhage of an artery into the brain.[4] Stroke is the third leading cause of death in the United States and a principal cause of disability in middle-aged and elderly people. The primary signal of a stroke is a sudden, temporary weakness or numbness of the face, arm, and/or leg on one side of the body. Other signals include temporary loss of speech or trouble speaking or understanding speech; temporary dimness or loss of vision, particularly in one eye; and unexplained dizziness, unsteadiness, or sudden falls. Sometimes major strokes are preceded by temporary attacks—"little strokes" whose symptoms are similar to those of a major stroke except that they last for only a very short time. Temporary attacks can occur days, weeks, or months before a severe stroke, so they should be taken seriously as warning signals. Prompt medical or surgical attention to these symptoms may prevent a major stroke.

Happily, the incidence of stroke has declined in recent years, and scientists at the National Institutes of Health believe that the drop is due to better control of high blood pressure through earlier diagnosis, medication, and dietary changes. In fact, that is why the FDA, in 1985, instituted a campaign to have the amount of salt in processed foods reduced. Labels now are supposed to inform you how much sodium is present in the package.

A teaspoon of table salt contains 2,000 milligrams of sodium, about 40 percent of its bulk. But sodium comes from many other sources, including from other ingredients added to foods. Baking soda is sodium bicarbonate. Often times vitamin C, which is called ascorbic acid, is added to food as sodium ascorbate. Monosodium glutamate (MSG) is about 10 percent sodium. Soy sauce is "liquid salt" at 1,099 milligrams per teaspoon. Some foods are naturally higher in sodium than others. For example, chard has 72 milligrams and spinach 49 milligrams of sodium per portion, while one ear of corn and a half cup of lima beans have only 1 milligram of sodium each.

Sodium, like sugar, may appear under a variety of names. Ingredients with sodium in the name, such as sodium bicarbonate and sodium ascorbate, are salty.

The National Academy of Sciences recommends that we ingest no more than 1,100 to 3,000 milligrams of sodium per day. The average American ingests 5,000 to 7,000 mg. If the numbers for sodium look very low on a label, look again and be aware of the difference between milligrams and grams. Some companies make you think there is less by saying only 5 grams of sodium, for example, which is really 5,000 milligrams.

The FDA does have established regulations for listing sodium on the label:

- Sodium free = less than 5 milligrams per serving

- Very low sodium = 35 milligrams or less per serving

- Low sodium = 140 milligrams or less per serving

- Reduced sodium = processed to reduce the usual level of sodium by 75 percent

- Unsalted = processed without salt

"No salt added" signifies that the producer didn't put any additional salt in during processing, but the food itself may still be naturally high in sodium.

The basic sources of cereals—wheat, corn, rice, and oats—are salt-free. Yet instant oatmeal contains about 360 milligrams, instant corn grits 590 milligrams, and instant cream of wheat 180 milligrams per serving. If you're willing to take the time to cook the whole-grain cereals, then you can avoid the high salt. It's providing the "instant" that dishes out the sodium.

Cold cereals are a matter of taste. Cheerios cereal, for example, one of the most popular for children, has 290 milligrams per serving. Wheaties cereal has 370 milligrams. Total cereal, which is really the same as Wheaties but with less salt, contains 290 milligrams of sodium. Shredded wheat has no salt.

It is a matter of choice, but sometimes it's hard to win. Food producers may lower one dietary ingredient while raising another. A *Consumer Reports* test showed that Borden's Wise Lite-Line chips and puffs contain 7 grams of fat and 140 calories per one-ounce serving, compared to the regular chips with 11 grams of fat and 160 calories. But the Wise Lite-Line chips has almost 175 milligrams of sodium per serving while the regular chips has only 120 milligrams. Low-fat puffed cheese curls contain only 5 grams of fat and 130 calories, compared to Cheese Doodles' 10 grams of fat and 150 calories. However, the low-fat puffs are sprinkled with 310 milligrams of salt, compared to the Doodles' 190 milligrams.[5]

Some researchers have suggested that the high sodium intake of adults is the result of acquiring a taste for sodium through the exposure to high-sodium foods during childhood.[6] On page 94 are some foods that are frequently eaten by children, with the sodium content per serving noted.

How to Lower Your Salt Intake.   Food producers are putting out more and more lower-salt products, so choose those over the regular variety when feasible. Avoid the following:

• Fast-food entrées (most are loaded with salt)

• Salted or smoked fish (rinse any fish before use, because markets store the fish on salted ice)

• Most frozen dinners

• Cheeses, except for the low-sodium types

• Pizza

• Pickled or packed-in-brine vegetables, such as "garden salads" and sauerkraut

	SERVING SIZE	SODIUM CONTENT (milligrams)
Wise potato chips	1 ounce	240
Fritos barbecue flavor corn chips	1 ounce	245
Cheetos cheese snacks	1 ounce	260
Mr. Salty pretzels	5½ pieces	685
Kellogg's Corn Flakes cereal	1¼ cup	305
Kix cereal	1½ cup	315
Cheerios cereal	1¼ cup	330
Wheaties cereal	1 cup	370
Oatmeal cookies	3	200
Fudge brownie	1	76–108
Chocolate chip cookies	1	30–110
Devil's food cake	¹⁄₁₂th	405
Chocolate ice cream	1 scoop	80–122
Vanilla ice cream	1 scoop	60–110
Frankfurter	1	378–620
McDonald's Big Mac hamburger	1	979
Pizza Hut pizza	½ 10-inch pie	1,431

- Condiments such as garlic salt (use garlic powder instead), chili sauce and catsup (use low-sodium versions), meat tenderizers, flavor enhancers such as MSG, prepared mustards (use low-sodium versions), and soy sauce (use lower-sodium version, which is still high in salt)

- Canned soups (except low-sodium versions)

- Some canned vegetables (check the labels for sodium content)

Not everyone is affected by salt. The American Heart Association's *Cardiovascular Research Report* announced recently that an Indiana University group had developed tests to determine just who is salt-sensitive and who is salt-resistant. Myron Weinberger, M.D., and his colleagues reported the group's results at the September 1986 meeting of the American Heart Association's Council on High Blood Pressure Research in Cleveland. Based on Dr. Weinberger's research, 40 to 50 percent of the estimated 57.7 million Americans with high blood pressure may be sensitive to salt.[7]

Subjects in the study were put on a low-salt diet and then given a salt solution intravenously, followed by an oral diuretic to remove the water. Researchers measured blood pressure after the subjects were given the salt water and again after it was eliminated. Those who had a drop in blood pressure of ten or more points after the diuretic were defined as salt-sensitive. Those who had a drop of five or less points were not considered salt-sensitive.

Dr. Weinberger found that 51 percent of those with high blood pressure and even 26 percent of the normal volunteers were salt-sensitive. Thirty-three percent of those in the high blood pressure group were not salt-sensitive, while 58 percent of the normal volunteers were not salt-sensitive.

A second test was done to determine whether normal people would have a drop in blood pressure on a low-sodium diet. At the end of three months, researchers found a significant reduction in blood pressure in both the teenagers and the adults with normal blood pressure.

Studies have shown that psychological stress can also cause sodium retention in humans, but only among persons at risk for developing high blood pressure who are also "hot responders." Their nervous systems are highly reactive to psychological stress.[8] It is Dr. Weinberger's belief that those who are salt-sensitive will eventually develop high blood pressure. If future studies prove this to be correct, it may be that the people identified as salt-sensitive can postpone high blood pressure by reducing the salt in their diet. Since hypertension is the leading cause of stroke, if high blood pressure can be controlled by diet alone, then perhaps you can prevent the conditions that set the stage for stroke.

In another study, a four-year trial assessed whether people with less severe high blood pressure could even discontinue antihypertensive drug therapy and use diet alone to control blood pressure. Rose Stamler, M.A., Jeremiah Stamler, M.D., and others of the Department of Community Health and Preventive Medicine at Northwestern University Medical School, Chicago, divided high blood pressure patients into three groups.[9] Participants were men and women, thirty-five years of age and older, who were receiving drugs for the treatment of high blood pressure. They were randomly assigned to one of three groups: (1) nutritional intervention throughout the trial, with withdrawal of high blood pressure medicine; (2) no nutritional intervention and discontinuation of medication; and (3) no nutritional intervention and continued therapy with high blood pressure medication. The patients in groups one and two were put back on drugs if their blood pressure rose too high.

In group one, loss of at least ten pounds was maintained by 30 percent of the group, with a mean loss of four pounds. Sodium intake fell 36 percent in group one, where alcohol was limited to two drinks a day or less. Fat was reduced from 39 percent to 32 percent and carbohydrates increased from 38 percent to 44 percent. At four years, 39 percent of the participants in group one had blood pressure that remained normal without drug therapy, compared with 5 percent of the participants in group two.

The researchers concluded from the findings that nutritional therapy may substitute for medication in a sizeable portion of those with high blood pressure. Or, if drugs are still needed, diet can lessen some of the unwanted side-effects of drug treatment such as gout, impotence, and malaise.

CHOLESTEROL AND YOUR BRAIN

Sending blood to the brain under pressure is a prime risk factor for stroke. The result may be a hemorrhage into the brain. A second risk factor is narrowed arteries that may become clogged.

If the stroke damage is to the right hemisphere of the brain, the left side of the body may be paralyzed, there may be difficulty in perceiving space, and the person may become impulsive and suffer memory deficits in performing movements. If the left side is damaged, there may be paralysis of the right side, speech and language deficits, and the person may become slow, cautious, and have difficulty remembering words.

There are countless studies in progress to correlate diet and stroke prevention. A great many of them involve a waxy alcohol called cholesterol that's found in everyone's living tissue. You need some cholesterol, and you get it in two ways. First, your body automatically manufactures most of the cholesterol it needs. Second, you increase your cholesterol levels by eating foods that contain it or that stimulate your body to increase its production. In the body, cholesterol is carried by three types of proteins. Two of them—low-density and very low density lipoprotein (LDL and VDL), which are composed of 50 percent or more cholesterol—seem to get caught in channels and clog arteries. The third type of protein, high-density lipoprotein (HDL) is considered the "good one." Consisting of about 20 to 25 percent cholesterol, HDL's carry off their cholesterol burden so that it can be disposed of by the body. Many researchers believe that HDL's are protective and that the ratio of HDL's to VDL's and LDL's in the blood is more important than the overall cholesterol count. Not everyone agrees with this theory, but most experts do advise that lowering saturated fat in the diet is a way of lowering cholesterol.

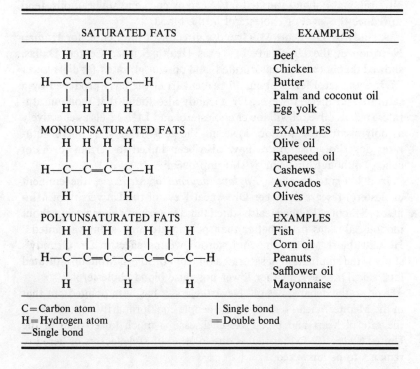

SATURATED FATS	EXAMPLES
H H H H | | | | H—C—C—C—C—H | | | | H H H H	Beef Chicken Butter Palm and coconut oil Egg yolk
MONOUNSATURATED FATS	EXAMPLES
H H H H | | | | H—C—C=C—C—H | | H H	Olive oil Rapeseed oil Cashews Avocados Olives
POLYUNSATURATED FATS	EXAMPLES
H H H H H H H | | | | | | | H—C—C=C—C—C=C—C—H | | | H H H	Fish Corn oil Peanuts Safflower oil Mayonnaise

C = Carbon atom | Single bond
H = Hydrogen atom   =Double bond
— Single bond

Fats are composed of carbon, hydrogen, and oxygen. They can be liquid or solid, depending on the type of fatty acids. Food fats are made up of three types of fatty acids that influence cholesterol levels in your blood: saturated, monounsaturated, and polyunsaturated. Highly saturated fats are usually animal fats. With the exception of a few vegetable fats such as palm and coconut oils, they are hard at room temperature and have the maximum number of hydrogen atoms attached to their carbon atoms (see chart on page 97). Saturated fats tend to raise blood levels of cholesterol.

Unsaturated fats, found mostly in plant foods, are short two or more hydrogen atoms, so they are usually liquid at room temperature. Unsaturated fats are further divided into two types: monounsaturated (two hydrogen atoms short of saturation) and polyunsaturated (four or more hydrogen atoms short of saturation). Monounsaturated fats, such as olive oil, and polyunsaturated fats, such as corn and soybean oils, tend to reduce the level of cholesterol in the blood.

A study by Dr. Scott M. Grundy, director of the Center for Human Nutrition at the University of Texas Health Science Center, Dallas, showed that both monounsaturated- and polyunsaturated-fat diets lower LDL cholesterol levels about 17 percent from the level produced by a saturated-fat diet. However, Dr. Grundy also found that monounsaturates such as olive oil will lower cholesterol and LDL levels as effectively as polyunsaturates, without lowering the good HDL's, as polyunsaturates do.[10] Polyunsaturates have also been linked to certain forms of cancer, although that link is still unproven.[11]

In a letter to the *New England Journal of Medicine,* the eminent cholesterol research pioneer Dr. Ancel Keys of the University of Minnesota School of Public Health stated that Dr. Grundy's conclusion about monounsaturates being better than polyunsaturates is "unwarranted." He said the reason for the cholesterol-lowering effect in Dr. Grundy's study is the elimination of saturated fat from the diets. Monounsaturated fats, said Dr. Keys, neither lower nor raise blood cholesterol.[12]

And so the debate goes on. Nevertheless, it has been pointed out that in the Mediterranean region, where people cook primarily with olive oil, the rate of heart and blood vessel disease is much lower than in the United States.[13] Whether that is due to other lifestyle factors or heredity remains to be answered.

As of this writing, no rules exist to protect consumers from product claims about saturated fats or cholesterol, although the FDA is in the process of forming a set of regulations. According to the agency's proposal, the following should be in the package when claims of lower cholesterol are on the label:

- Cholesterol-free = less than 2 milligrams per serving
- Low cholesterol = less than 20 milligrams per serving

In addition to keeping the arteries unclogged by fat, researchers are seeking to prevent blood clots from forming and blocking arteries. Among the studies in progress are those involving garlic and fish oil.

An international team of scientists has synthesized a potent new anticlotting agent from garlic.[14] This new compound is made from a garlic chemical that has medical value as an antibiotic. That chemical is *allicin,* which forms only when a garlic clove is cut or cooked. It has long been known to promote wound healing but is also recognized as a skin irritant.

James L. Catalfamo, Ph.D., a blood specialist at the New York State Department of Health, says that potentially, the garlic derivative could lead to therapies for people at risk for stroke, heart attack, and hardening of the arteries. It also appears to be more specific than aspirin, which should allow a more controlled therapy with fewer side-effects. The new compound prevents the first step in the clotting process—the clumping of platelets, the blood cells responsible for clotting. Aspirin works later in the process and in a more general way.[15]

Omega-3 fish oil also prevents platelets from clotting. The linking of fish oil and the maintenance of healthy blood vessels began in the 1970s, when Danish researchers discovered that Eskimos living in Greenland and who consumed 40 percent of their calories from animal fat, had a much lower rate of heart attack than would be expected from such a high-fat diet.[16] It wasn't because Eskimos were genetically immune to fat-clogged arteries, the scientist observed, because those Eskimos who adopted a typical American or European diet soon developed the same rate of heart disease as citizens of those continents.

As the research progressed, the Danes observed that Eskimos bruised more easily. The scientists pursued this clue and found the reason for the black-and-blue marks: the Eskimos' platelets, which float in blood and help with clotting, were less "sticky" than those typically in the blood of Americans and Europeans. This suggested that the arteries of Greenland Eskimos were being protected by something that alters the way their platelets function. That something turned out to be the omega-3 fatty acids derived from cold-water fish.

Other studies have confirmed the Greenland discovery. In one research project, for example, Dutch investigators, who followed 852 men for twenty years, reported that those who ate more than one ounce of fish daily were half as likely to have a heart attack as the men who rarely ate fish.[17]

Fish oils—primarily eicosapentaenoic acid or omega-3 fatty acids— are not without side effects. Fish oil has been found to affect blood clotting and cause easy bruising; its long-term effects are uncertain. Doctors persuaded by fish oil benefits, however, are now recommending that high-risk patients eat more fish, particularly dark-meat, deep-water fish.

The current research points to the following conclusion: if you eat cold-water fish with lots of garlic cooked in olive oil without salt, you will help to protect your brain against a stroke.

FISH OIL SOURCES

EXCELLENT	GOOD
Codliver oil	Lobster*
Mackerel	Crab
Salmon	Hake
Bluefish	Shark
Herring	Oyster
Mullet	
Sardines	
Tuna	

*A substance in shellfish wrongly identified as cholesterol by a food chemist has led to it being labeled as being imprudent in a low-cholesterol diet. The *Harvard Medical School Health Letter* (February 1986) points out that shellfish is low in cholesterol, and does have the beneficial fish oil, and is a good substitute for red meat.

⧊ 6 ⧊

The Allergy/Brain/Behavior Connection

I s it something you're eating that makes you irritable?

The early Greek physician and philosopher Hippocrates was one of the first to note that cow's milk could cause health problems for some people. The actual number of people who are allergic to cow's milk or any other offender is unknown. The effect of food allergy on the brain is even more difficult to determine.

Some immunologists and psychiatrists are convinced that allergy plays a part in a number of brain disorders, including depression, schizophrenia, Alzheimer's disease, hyperactivity, and autism. There are even more experts who believe that allergies have nothing to do with these disorders. No one knows for certain, but we will describe some of the intriguing current theories and research. One thing no one can deny is that if you suffer from an allergy of any sort, the discomfort can affect your brain, mood, and behavior.

An *adverse reaction* or sensitivity to a food means *any abnormal* reaction to a food or food additive that is eaten, whether caused by allergic or nonallergic mechanisms. It is important to distinguish between an *allergy* and an *intolerance*.

- **Food sensitivities** (allergic reactions) involve the body's defensive immune system.

- **Food intolerances** do not involve the immune system.

The following are adverse reactions to food that are often mistakenly believed to be allergic reactions:

- **Food Intolerance:** an adverse reaction to food due to such factors as enzyme deficiencies, contaminants or toxins, drug use, heredity, psychological disorder, or underlying disease. If you get indigestion from eating beans, that's an intolerance. The adverse reaction is usually caused by factors in the diet other than protein. One of the more common food intolerance reactions may be the result of the body's inability to digest lactose (milk sugar). Many people, particularly as they grow older, have this "lactose intolerance." They are deficient in the enzyme needed to process lactose.

- **Pharmacologic Food Reaction:** an adverse reaction to a chemical found in a food or food additive that produces a druglike effect, such as caffeine in coffee causing the "jitters" or the amines in cheese causing a headache.

  The "Chinese restaurant syndrome," manifested by anxiety, flushed face, and pressure in the chest, has been shown to be caused by eating large amounts of the flavor enhancer MSG. Sulfite preservatives are now known to have the potential to cause a serious attack of asthma and even death.

- **Food Poisoning:** an adverse reaction caused by a food or food additive without your immune system being involved. Toxins (poisons or bacteria) may be either contained within the food or released by microorganisms or parasites contaminating the food (see chapter 8).

Food allergy, on the other hand, involves the immune system. If you are allergic to a food or food additive, your body's immune system overreacts to it. The food or food additive may be harmless to others, but you suffer irritating, uncomfortable symptoms because you are hypersensitive to it. The word *allergy* is derived from two Greek words that can be roughly translated as "altered response."

The National Institute of Allergy and Infectious Diseases estimates that there are thirty-five-million people in this country who have allergic reactions to substances that, in similar amounts, are apparently completely harmless to most people. The number of ailments diagnosed as allergies is undoubtedly going to rise as more and more is discovered about this group of diseases and as our environment becomes more and more complex.

A turning point in the field of allergy occurred in 1967 at the Children's Asthma Research Institute and Hospital in Denver. Drs. Kimishige and Teruko Ishizaka—a husband and wife team of scientists supported by the National Institute of Allergy and Infectious Diseases—discovered the antibody now known as *immunoglobulin E* (IgE) which is responsible for most allergic reactions. The substances that cause allergic reactions are *allergens* and *antigens*. If you are allergic, the first time you encountered an allergen, your body made millions of IgE antibodies against it. The IgE antibodies then became bound to two types of cells in your body—the basophils in your blood and the mast cells found primarily in your skin and the tissues of your respiratory and digestive tracts. When you again encountered the same allergen, it attached to the IgE antibodies already bound to your basophils and mast cells. This combination of allergen and IgE then signals your basophils and mast cells to release *histamine,* which comes from cells in the connective tissues, especially beneath the mucous membranes and the skin, and *bradykinin,* which is found in blood plasma. Histamine can cause swelling of the mucous membranes in the nose and itching of the eyes. Bradykinin can contract the smooth muscle of the walls of the small tubes in the lungs. This sequence of events does not necessarily occur when something you eat "doesn't agree with you."

It is very difficult to recognize a food allergy because:

- Allergic reactions may be delayed from several hours to days after ingestion of the offending food.

- You may eat the food only once in awhile.

- There may be hidden additives and contaminants in the food.

- You may be allergic to that food only at certain times.

- There may be an interaction between a food and a drug you are taking.

- The quantity of food eaten may influence the reaction.

- The cooking method may influence the reaction.

Symptoms of delayed sensitivity may include anything from muscle aches to mental symptoms, drowsiness, and confusion, all of which are also symptoms of many other, nonallergic ailments.

There is no doubt, however, about a food allergy when an anaphylactic attack occurs. It is an immediate, dramatic, life-threatening, generalized allergic reaction. It may involve any system of the body but usually affects the skin, nose, throat, lungs, stomach, heart, and blood vessels. The first signs may be a red, itchy rash and a feeling of warmth. These may be followed by light-headedness, shortness of breath or sneezing, a feeling of anxiety, stomach or uterine cramps, and/or vomiting and diarrhea. Foods frequently listed as the causes of anaphylaxis include peanuts, nuts, shellfish, eggs, and seeds.

Food allergens are usually proteins. The fact that neurotransmitters in the brain are made from proteins suggests that brain allergies may exist. Most of the allergens can still cause reactions even after they have undergone digestion. Recent studies in the United States indicate that proteins in cow's milk, eggs, peanuts, wheat, and soy are the most common food allergens.[2] Other common food allergens include shellfish, pork, corn, strawberries, tuna, chicken, chocolate, nuts, tomatoes, peas, oranges, and cabbage. But almost any food can be an allergen. Also, some people can become sensitive to the artificial coloring agents, vegetable gums, and other substances widely used in prepared foods. Cooking can reduce the effect of some protein allergens but may increase the effect of others.[3]

Sometimes an allergen is a food that has been eaten for many years without any ill effect. Unknown to the victim, the allergy has been developing slowly. If symptoms of a food allergy appear quickly—during a meal or just after a specific food has been eaten—it is usually fairly easy to discover the responsible allergen. But if the reaction is delayed, then it is necessary to investigate by the process of elimination, excluding a few foods at a time from the diet to see whether symptoms are relieved; or by the technique of challenge—that is, by initially giving a limited diet to which other foods are gradually added, one at a time, until symptoms appear. If the allergy is mild, it may never be possible to pinpoint the food allergen.

Skin tests are generally of little value in diagnosing food allergies. Also, other conditions in the stomach and intestines that may be quite serious can cause symptoms that mimic food allergy. A careful history is the best diagnostic tool. You could help your physician and yourself detect a food allergy, if it exists, by using the chart on page 105.

In some food groups, especially legumes and seafoods, an allergy to one member of the food group may result in your being allergic to some

INSTRUCTIONS: List each food once down the left side of the chart. Use a *B* for breakfast, an *L* for lunch, a *D* for dinner, and an *O* for other to indicate when you ate the food. If symptoms occurred, put an *X* over the letter. For example, if you ate tuna for lunch on Wednesday, you'd list tuna, mark an *L* under Wednesday, and, if symptoms occurred, put an *X* over the *L*. In the diary at the bottom of the chart, record the food that caused the symptom, the date the symptom occurred, and under what circumstance, and a description of the symptoms. For example, Wednesday, week 1, write: Tuna. Lunch at a restaurant. Developed a headache.

WEEK 1
DATE:
FOOD S / M / T / W / T / F / S

DATE: _____ FOOD EATEN: _____
SYMPTOMS: _____

WEEK 2
DATE:
FOOD: S / M / T / W / T / F / S

_____ CIRCUMSTANCES: _____

other member in the same group. This is known as *cross-reactivity*. Persons allergic to peanuts, for example, are more likely to be allergic to soybeans, peas, and other legumes than to walnuts or pecans. However, some people may be allergic to both peanuts and walnuts. These allergies are called *coincidental allergies*.

Some children's specific food allergies may disappear completely as they mature. If a food causes an allergic reaction in an adult, however, it must usually be dropped from the diet permanently. This means all forms of the allergen—for example, a person allergic to eggs may have to avoid eating prepared foods that contain eggs, such as cakes, custards, and waffles. He also may have to forego certain protective immunizations, like the influenza vaccine.

Since we are concerned with food and the brain, let's get to the most commonly accepted food/brain/allergy connection: the headache. When you have a headache, it is not actually your brain that aches but rather it is the blood vessels in and around your brain that are producing the pain. However, when your head aches, you can't use your brain efficiently.

APPLE FAMILY	BIRCH FAMILY	BUCKWHEAT FAMILY
Apples	Filberts	Buckwheat
Pears	Hazelnuts	Rhubarb
Quinces	Wintergreen	
Vinegar		
CASHEW FAMILY	CITRUS FAMILY	GINGER FAMILY
Cashews	Grapefruit	Cardamom
Mangos	Kumquats	Ginger
Pistachios	Lemons	Tumeric
	Limes	
	Oranges	
	Tangerines	
GOOSEBERRY FAMILY	GOOSEFOOT FAMILY	GOURD FAMILY
Currants	Beets	Casaba melon
Gooseberries	Spinach	Cucumbers
	Swiss chard	Honeydew melon
		Muskmelon
		Persian melon
		Pumpkin
		Squash
		Watermelon

GRAINS
Barley
Bran
Cellulose
Corn
Dextrose
Glucose
Gluten flour
Graham flour
Malt
Molasses
Oats
Rice
Sorghum
Sugar cane
Wheat and wheat germ

GRAPE FAMILY
Cream of Tartar
Grapes
Raisins

HEATH FAMILY
Blueberries
Cranberries

LAUREL FAMILY
Avocados
Bay leaves
Cinnamon

LEGUMES
Acacia
Black-eyed peas
Kidney beans
Lentils
Licorice
Lima beans
Navy beans
Peanuts
Peas
Sennas
Soybeans
String beans

LILY FAMILY
Aloe
Asparagus
Chives
Garlic
Leeks
Onions

MINT FAMILY
Marjoram
Mint
Peppermint
Sage
Savory
Spearmint
Thyme

**MORNING GLORY
FAMILY**
Sweet potatoes

**MULBERRY
FAMILY**
Breadfruit
Fig
Hops
Mulberries

MUSTARD FAMILY
Broccoli
Brussels sprouts
Cabbage
Cauliflower
Mustard
Rutabagas
Turnips

MYRTLE FAMILY
Allspice
Cloves
Guava
Paprika
Pimento

OLIVE FAMILY
Green olives
Olive oil
Ripe olives

ORCHID FAMILY
Vanilla

PALM FAMILY
Coconuts
Dates
Sago

PARSLEY FAMILY
Cabbage
Carrots
Celery
Collard greens
Horseradish
Kale
Kohlrabies
Parsley
Parsnip
Radishes
Watercress

PINE FAMILY
Juniper

PLUM FAMILY
Almonds
Apricots
Cherries
Nectarines
Peaches
Plums
Prunes

POTATO FAMILY
Cayenne
Chile
Eggplant
Green peppers
Potatoes
Red peppers
Tomatoes

ROSE FAMILY
Blackberries
Dewberries
Loganberries
Raspberries
Strawberries

**SUNFLOWER
  FAMILY**
Jerusalem artichokes
Sunflower seeds

WALNUT FAMILY
Anise
Butternuts
Caraway
Coriander
Dill
Fennel
Hickory nuts
Pecans
Walnuts

CAN HEADACHES BE DUE TO A FOOD ALLERGY?

About half of all patients seen by family physicians mention headaches as a symptom. There are several types of headaches and also several causes. A hypersensitive reaction to food protein could trigger an attack. One example is the mold-sensitive adult who also has migraines and who eats mold-containing foods.[4] One particular form of headache is the *migraine* (literally, "half the skull"), which some surveys say affects 10 percent of all Americans. It is generally agreed now that migraines are allergic in origin. The most common allergens include eggs, milk, chocolate, and pork.

As its name implies, migraines are often confined to one side of the head. The "classic" migraine consists of a forewarning, or *prodromal,* such a flashing lights or flickering vision followed by an initially throbbing or pulsating headache that later becomes steady or dull. However, most migraines are not classic, and experts increasingly use the phrase "migraine variants" to cover the other kinds of headaches and associated symptoms like nausea and vomiting. For example, "cluster headaches"—so called because they tend to occur in clusters over a period of days, weeks, or months—are probably part of the migraine family. Some headaches that formerly were labeled as "sinus headaches," because of the accompanying stuffy nose and pain in the sinus area, are now recognized as migraines. The common underlying factor for all of the headaches labeled migraine is the role played by the blood vessels of the neck and head. There is solid evidence that symptoms that occur just before the headache strikes are usually related to the constriction of these vessels and that the actual headache occurs when these vessels subsequently expand. The exact reason for these blood vessel changes are not certain, although current interest is focused on the role of platelets and brain neurotransmitters such as serotonin.[5] Diet is certainly a big factor. Changes in pattern such as fasting or missing meals, specific foods, excessive caffeine, or sudden withdrawal from caffeine, liquor, food preservatives such as nitrites, flavor enhancers such as MSG, and even salt have been implicated as causes.

In September 1984, the British medical journal *Lancet* described a test in which patients with a history of migraine headaches had meals containing egg, milk, and wheat (foods known to produce symptoms in these patients). The test confirmed that migraine in these particular cases was an allergic response.[6]

During the late 1960s, British and Danish physicians pinpointed two major abnormalities that underlie migraine headaches: (1) a decrease in blood flow through the brain before the headache, and (2) an increase in blood flow through the brain during the headache.[7]

Scientists are now discovering why these blood flow changes occur. They suspect the neurotransmitter serotonin and the mast cells. The level of serotonin, a number of researchers have noted, rises suddenly in the blood just before a headache hits and is believed to cause the pre-headache symptoms of numbness, partial paralysis, and "flashing lights" that many migraine sufferers experience. According to current theory, the level of serotonin then drops, and the constricted blood vessels pop open, dilate, and the pounding headache hits.

Evidence for this theory was gained when twenty patients were given the drug Nardil, which prevents the breakdown of serotonin in the blood. Seven of the patients became virtually headache-free, seven suffered only one-fourth the number of pretreatment attacks, and six suffered half as many as before.[8]

As far as the mast cells are concerned, they attach themselves to the surface of antigens and are the prime cells in the body that produce histamine. That is why we take antihistamines to combat allergies. Histamine, serotonin, and bradykinin, which stimulates the mucous glands, have long been known to play a part in allergy and are now clearly implicated in migraine for three reasons:

1. They can constrict smooth muscle.

2. They can dilate tiny blood vessels.

3. They can stimulate pain receptors.

Such actions are part of the vascular, painful, and mind-stopping features of migraine attacks.

Dietary factors such as changes in pattern (fasting or missing meals) and specific foods may directly or indirectly cause the release of these three culprits—histamine, serotonin, and bradykinin. The suspected foods and their ingredient "triggers" are listed here.

FOODS THAT MAY CAUSE HEADACHES	
Cheese	Tryptophan and tyramine
Chocolate and cocoa	Dopamine and phenylethylamine
Red wine	Tyramine
Herring	Tyramine and salt
Alcohol	Histamine
Tomatoes	Histamine
Coffee	Caffeine
Chocolate	Theobromine
Colas	Caffeine
Tea	Caffeine and theobromine
Oranges and other citrus fruits	Histamine
Cured meats	Nitrates and nitrites
Flavor enhancers	MSG and salt

TENSION-FATIGUE SYNDROME

The term *tension-fatigue syndrome* refers to alternating periods of anxiety and listlessness associated with allergic diseases. As early as 1922, W. R. Shannon described the cases of eight children suffering from a variety of behavior complaints such as extreme nervousness, irritability, unruliness, insomnia, decreased appetite, and poor school performance. He believed that of these children's complaints were due to irritation of the nervous system by allergic reactions. Because marked improvement in seven of the eight patients was reported upon the elimination of certain foods from the diet, he suggested that food proteins were common triggers of such reactions.[9] In 1954, Dr. F. Speer enlarged on the observations and said that the behavior of affected children seemed to have two contributing facets:

1. Tension was manifested by hyperactivity, restlessness, emotional instability, and insomnia.

2. Fatigue was evidenced by listlessness and constant tiredness that was not made better by resting.[10]

HYPERACTIVITY BY ANY OTHER NAME AND DIET

Hyperactivity, attention-deficit disorder, or tension-fatigue syndrome—depending on who is referring to the constellation of behavior—may be caused by anxiety, a physical ailment, or the environment, or it may be strictly in the eyes of the beholder.

The prevalence of the syndrome is not clear, but it has been estimated to involve between 5 and 10 percent of American schoolchildren.

The possible relationship between attention-deficit disorder with hyperactivity and natural salicylates as well as other food additives was presented by Benjamin Feingold, a California physician, in 1973. On the basis of experience in treating adult patients with aspirin intolerance, Dr. Feingold promoted a theory that hyperactive behavior and learning disorders in children might be the result of a reaction to natural salicylates in certain foods. Later, because of the known cross-reactivity between aspirin and tartrazine, Food, Drug and Cosmetic Act (FD & C) Yellow Dye no. 5, all food colorings were suspected as offenders. Still later, the preservatives sodium benzoate and BHA/BHT were incriminated. A regimen called the Kaiser Permanente Diet or Feingold Diet was popularized by Dr. Feingold in a book on the subject.[11] The special diet, devoid of foods suspected of having not only significant levels of natural salicylates but also food coloring and preservatives, was alleged to produce improvement in 50 percent of the patients with hyperactivity and attention deficits. For more information about the Feingold Diet, see pages 134–138.

The controversy concerning the link between food allergies and hyperactive behavior continues, as do debates over a number of other brain/behavior/allergy links.

THE DEPRESSION/ALLERGY CONNECTION

What role does allergy play in the "blues"? In tests of depressed patients, the percentage of those with allergies ranged from 33 to 70 percent, compared to two percent in controls.[12]

The apparently high incidence of "allergy" in depression requires further study, according to John W. Crayton, M.D., associate professor of psychiatry at the University of Chicago. He points out that the medications widely used to treat depression today, tricyclic antidepressants, are potent antihistamines, and that the same histamine-controlled reactions in allergy might also be involved in certain depressions. A recent observation that aids evidence to the allergy/depression connection is that the gene associated with depression lies on chromosome 6, near the genes involved in the immune response. The clinical significance of this finding in relation to adverse reactions to foods remains to be determined.

THE SCHIZOPHRENIA/ALLERGY CONNECTION

The link between schizophrenia, the most common type of psychosis, and allergy may be even more intangible than that of allergy and depression, and yet there are some intriguing connections.

The prime suspect has been a common allergen, wheat. The first clue emanates from epidemiological studies. It has been noticed that in populations that do not have wheat in their diet, schizophrenia is also absent. The second clue is that patients with schizophrenia seem to have more allergies than people who are not schizophrenic but are suffering from other mental disorders.

Experts of the Schizophrenia Association of Great Britain emphasize milk allergy in their literature. A gluten protein, *alpha gliadin,* which is purified from wheat flour, is active against nerve tissue. The same amino acid sequence found in alpha gliadin also has been found in casein, the major protein in milk. The clinical significance, if any, of these findings is unknown.[13]

In a 1982 study published in *Psychological Medicine,* British researchers reported their attempt to test the validity of the food allergy theory of schizophrenia by measuring antibodies to wheat, milk, and other dietary protein in a group of schizophrenic patients and their close relatives who were not affected by the illness.[14]

A total of thirty-six out of ninety-eight patients had antibodies in their blood to one or more of the substances tested. In fifteen of these there was only a weakly positive reaction. Two of the thirty-six had significantly higher food antibodies.

The researchers noted that while only two of the patients had significantly higher food antibody reactions, the patients had a greater number of minor reactions to the antibodies tested, particularly to certain cow proteins, and a higher overall level of antibodies in their blood than the ninety relatives who served as controls.

The British researchers feel that tranquilizers the patients were taking may have thrown off the test results by showing patients to be more allergic than they actually were. The investigators concluded, however, that their study cast serious doubt over the food allergy/schizophrenia connection for the majority of schizophrenics, since high levels of food antibodies were found in only two of the thirty-eight subjects. However, they added, there is a suggestion that schizophrenic patients may be more susceptible than their normal relatives to a variety of allergens.

AUTISM AND ALLERGY

Also in 1982, researchers in Israel reported a study of autistic children at the Geha Psychiatric Hospital in Petah Tiqva.[15] The investigators found that the brains of these youngsters may be misperceiving a basic brain protein as a foreign body and, as a result, systematically destroying it through an allergic reaction. The resulting brain damage, although undetectable, may be responsible for the constellation of emotional, intellectual, and social handicaps that characterize the disorder. Autistic children have an inability to form meaningful interpersonal relationships.

ALZHEIMER'S AND ALLERGY

Alzheimer's disease, that brain-degenerating, memory-destroying condition afflicting mostly older adults, is also suspected of being linked to a brain allergy. Autopsies on its victims show that there are "dead spots" on the nerves in their brains composed of tangles of nerve fibers and deposits of waste material. Researchers at Albert Einstein Medical Center in New York took material from the brains of Alzheimer's victims at autopsy and extracted antigens from it. They found that the antigens reacted with brain tissue from other Alzheimer's victims but not with that from people who had died from other causes. This led Einstein investigators to conclude that there is an "antigen-antibody" reaction involved in Alzheimer's, since the brain tissue from Alzheimer's victims was highly selective for that of other Alzheimer's patients.[16]

Such research reports are intriguing, but the question of whether a brain allergy exists still has no definitive answer. Since allergic reactions can damage other organs, such as the lung and the skin, there is reason to believe that they may also injure the brain, despite the barriers nature has erected to protect it. The effects may be as devastating as Alzheimer's or as mild as an irritable mood.

MOOD AND FOOD ALLERGY

Dr. John Crayton of the University of Chicago is one researcher who has found a possible link between food and mood, but he is quick to point out the limitations of such findings.[17] In his study, a group of thirty-five volunteers—some with complaints of food sensitivity—were fed capsules of powdered wheat, milk, or chocolate, foods often associated with allergies. He found that changes in mood, coincidental with changes in the immune system, did occur in this group. He theorizes that food-induced reactions may cause local swelling in the brain that leads to mood swings, but cautions that this is early work and not yet understood.

Dr. Crayton points out that because of the widespread reports of food sensitivity producing behavioral effects, the question has been raised as to whether food could produce effects on the brain and behavior in the absence of effects on other body systems. He said a review of the case histories of several workers in this field suggest that individuals with food sensitivity with only brain and behavioral dysfunction must be extremely rare. In most studies, all of the subjects had both physical and mental symptoms.

The real problem, he said, is defining whether the allergic condition actually causes the behavioral symptoms on a physical basis or whether the emotional or behavioral symptoms are primarily psychological reactions to being physically ill.

Summing it up, the debate about food allergy has experts on one side explaining the commonly reported links between food allergy and behavior as:

1. Coincidental, because behavioral symptoms and allergy are both so common that they can often coexist in the same person.

2. Any chronic condition such as allergy can create emotional problems both in the victim and the victim's family and result in tension and fatigue.

3. Allergy may cause symptoms of wheezing, sneezing, itching, coughing, and shortness of breath which, in turn, may make you so uncomfortable or so upset that you are irritable and can't concentrate.

The experts on the other side say that brain allergy does exists and that it causes all sorts of emotional, behavioral, and physical problems.

There is no scientific proof of primary brain allergy, other than so-called anecdotal reports based mostly on the observations of family members, psychologists, and physicians. That does not mean that it doesn't exist, however, and it is certainly possible that a definitive link between food allergy and the brain will soon be uncovered.

In the meantime, there is only one way to "cure" a food allergy: avoid the offending substance. Here are some hints:

Keep a diary. You can help yourself and your physician identify the allergen by keeping a diary of *everything* you eat and drink for a week or two—that includes snacks, gum, and candy.

Keep a record of your symptoms. If you record your well-being or distress about an hour after you have eaten the meals and recorded the food in your diary, you will probably begin to make an association between something you ingested and your mental and physical symptoms of distress.

Buy foods without the offenders. Whether you have an allergy or a sensitivity, once you have identified the substances that bother you, you can obtain foods that are made without it. They may be more expensive, but you may like certain dishes and think them worth the extra cost. If you find you must avoid wheat, for example, or lactose, you can write to the following companies who produce a line of foods for the allergic or sensitive:

DIETARY SPECIALITIES, P.O. Box 227, Rochester, N.Y. 14601, provides wheat-free products, such as Aproten pastas, that are cornstarch-based. It also has wheat starch, barley mixes, and low-protein, low-sodium, low-calcium, and low-potassium canned breads, cookies and cake mixes. It offers brochures and recipes. The products are available in health food stores and by mail order.

ENER-G-FOODS, P.O. Box 84487, 6901 Fox Avenue South, Seattle, Wa. 98124-5787, produces and sells gluten-free, wheat-free, dairy-free and lactose-free products including a wide selection of breads (brown rice bread, white rice bread, tapioca, bread, etc), cookies, doughnuts, crackers, buns, rolls and mixes. These are vacuum packages for a six-month unrefrigerated shelflife.

Ener-G Foods offers a brochure and a complete listing of products and ingredients. Although the products are in health food stores and some supermarkets much of their business is done by mail order. Also available in Canada, in the U.K., Australia and Israel.

FEARN NATURAL FOODS, P.O. Box 09398, 3015 West Vera Avenue, Milwaukee, Wisc. 53209: gluten-free products include Fearn Soya products, Blackbean, and Falafel Mix. The following pancake mixes contain no dairy ingredients: Rich Earth, Buckwheat, Low Sodium, and Whole Wheat. Breakfast Patty Mix and Sunflower Burger Mix contain no wheat or dairy ingredients. The company's Liquid Lecithin (mint flavored) contains no gluten, wheat, or dairy ingredients. A number of free recipe booklets for the allergic are available. Just send a large stamped, self-addressed envelope. Products are available in health food stores and by mail order (by the case only).

GENERAL MILLS, 9200 Wayzata Boulevard, Minneapolis, Minn. 55440: corn-free products include granola bars, granola cereals, Cheerios cereal, and Wheathearts cereal. Lists of chocolate-free, wheat-free, milk-free and egg-free products are available.

GERBER PRODUCTS COMPANY, Department P.C., 445 South State Street, Fremont, Mich. 49412, has a number of gluten-free, corn-free, wheat-free, citrus-free, egg-free, and milk-free baby foods. You can write for special dietary sheets available for the allergic child or for a brochure for milk- , wheat- , egg- , or citrus-sensitive adults.

HAIN PUREFOOD COMPANY, 13660 South Figueroa, Los Angeles, Calif. 90061: egg-free mayonnaise and corn-free salad dressing made with safflower oil, milk-free safflower margarine, and some soups without corn or gluten are available in supermarkets and health food stores. The company will send recipes upon request, but their recipes are not specifically for the allergic.

HEINZ U.S.A., Consumer Relations Department, P.O. Box 57, Pittsburgh, Pa. 15230–0057, has milk- , wheat- , gluten- , egg- , and citrus-free products such as oatmeal and rice cereals with apples and bananas. Baby foods include gluten- , milk- , egg- , wheat- , and citrus-free products such as apples, pears, applesauce, and apricots, all fruit juices except orange juice and Orange-Apple-Banana Juice drinks, both of which contain citrus. Heinz has removed added salt from all varieties and added sweetener from all but tart fruits, desserts, and cereals.

Presently, there is no added sugar in 78 of their 112 products. Also, their baby foods do not contain artificial colors or flavors, preservatives, or flavor enhancers. You may write for the company's free booklet, *Planning Meals for the Allergic Infant,* or for a number of sheets with ingredient lists and the foods that may be appropriate for specific allergies.

LOMA LINDA FOODS, 11503 Pierce, Riverside, Calif. 92505, offers milk-free Soyagen for adults and Soyalac for infants, milk-free and corn-free l-soyalac for infants, wheat-free Nutina vegetable protein loaf, and Vitaburger. Nutina is also yeast-free. Many products free of eggs, artificial coloring and flavoring, MSG, wheat, corn, yeast, spices, caramel, dextrose, sucrose, and fructose. Not every product is free of all these items, but all are milk free. You can write to the company for a list of products and ingredients. Brochures are available for those products that can be used by the allergic or sensitive. Products are not sold by mail order but can be found in supermarkets and health food stores across the country.

◄ 7 ►

Food and Drug Interactions

T   hings had been going pretty badly for Charlie. His fur business was
    being affected by pickets in front of his store who wanted to prevent
    the slaughter of animals. Charlie, a short, balding, fifty-three-
year-old, didn't hunt or kill leopards or minks, he just sold coats, like his
father before him. To make matters worse, his eldest daughter was getting
a divorce and his youngest son was still "trying to find himself" at age
twenty-five.

An internist, knowing that Charlie was having a hard time, prescribed
an antidepressant. The medicine took effect, and about three weeks later
Charlie was feeling so well that he decided to take out his wife, Lillian,
for a celebration dinner. They went to their favorite restaurant. Charlie
ordered pickled herring for an appetizer and calf's liver and onions for the
main course, and he toasted Lillian with a glass of wine.

The furrier never made it home that night. He suffered a stroke. The
tyramine in the herring, liver, and wine raised his blood pressure and the
MAO-inhibitor in his medication prevented the enzyme from breaking
down the tyramine. When tyramine builds up, serious symptoms may
occur, including severe high blood pressure, excruciating headaches, nausea, and irregular heartbeat, within thirty to forty minutes after ingestion.
In Charlie's case, the buildup of tyramine made his blood pressure shoot
up. The increased pressure in his brain caused a weakened blood vessel to
blow like a worn tire, and he suffered a stroke. Fortunately, he had no
permanent disability. He recovered his appetite for life and no longer needs
the antidepressant. Herring and liver are no longer on his menu, however.
The former has too much salt and the latter too much cholesterol. Lillian
won't let him drink wine, because she blames it for his illness. So Charlie's
eating habits have really changed.

The severity of such an attack depends not only on how much tyramine there is in food but also on the dosage of the interacting medication and the physical size and health of the person ingesting the combination. The reaction would also depend on the brand of food and how long the products had been unrefrigerated. (The longer they are unrefrigerated, the higher the levels of amino acids.)

The interaction between MAO-inhibitors and tyramine-containing foods has been recognized since 1961, when it was first observed in patients receiving antidepressant drugs.[1]

The following are some recognized interactions between drugs and high-tyramine foods.

On the other hand, the tyramine food-drug combination that raises blood pressure can benefit people whose blood pressure drops too low when they stand up. Thirty-six-year-old Sandy, a homemaker and mother of three, suffered from positional hypotension. Every time she got out of bed or stood up from a chair, her blood pressure would suddenly drop; she would become dizzy and, on rare occasions, pass out. Her

DRUGS	HIGH-TYRAMINE FOODS	SYMPTOMS
MAO-Inhibitors	Cheese	Extreme high blood
Marplan	Beer	pressure
Norpramin	Wines	Heart palpitations
Parnate	Pickled herring	Vomiting
Nardil	Chicken liver	Flushing
	Yeast extract	Headaches
Anti-TB Drugs	Canned figs	Stroke
Isonazid and others	Raisins	Nausea
	Bananas	
Anti-cancer Drugs	Avocados	
Procarbazine	Chocolate	
Matulane	Soy sauce	
	Fava beans	
	Meat tenderizers	
	Eggplant	
	Tea	
	Cola	
	Liver	
	Yogurt	

physician prescribed a monoamine oxidase inhibitor drug and told Sandy to eat 90 grams of cheddar cheese—equivalent to 28 milligrams of tyramine—per day. She was then able to rise from a lying or sitting position without discomfort.[2]

Other food-drug interactions besides tyramine and MAO-inhibitors can be life threatening. Take Linda's case. Linda, a natural foods enthusiast, drank a lot of herbal tea. One day, after hurting her back while planting her vegetable garden, she took two tablets of the over-the-counter pain killer acetaminophen. She then injured her finger on a wire fence, and her husband had to take her to the emergency room because the minor cut wouldn't stop bleeding. It was apparently caused by the combination of the blood-thinning activity of the drug and the tea, which contained a natural derivative of the anti-blood-clotting agent, *coumarin.*

While Charlie's and Linda's cases were rather dramatic, most drug-food interactions are more subtle. Not every incompatibility is as obvious or as predictable. The seriousness and even the occurrence of food and drug interactions often depend on who you are: your heredity, weight, age, sex, and overall health. Some foods may clash directly with drugs; others lower, slow down, or magnify the amount of medication entering the bloodstream. In still other cases, the medication simply undercuts the normal nutrition (see chapter 00). First, let's consider how the interaction takes place.

Attallah Kappas, M.D., physician-in-chief at the Rockefeller University Hospital in New York, and Karl Anderson, M.D., traced the effects of everyday things we ingest, such as charcoal-broiled meats, broccoli, medications, and over-the-counter painkillers, and how such chemicals interact with each other.

The potency and duration of action of the chemicals ingested are determined in large part by the rate at which they are processed in our bodies. "If, for example, nothing were to happen to a drug after it entered your body and reached its target organ, it might continue to act indefinitely," Dr. Kappas explains. "However, most drugs are inactivated and excreted."[3]

Some drugs are transformed chemically in the intestine, some in the lungs, the kidneys, or the skin. By far, the greater number of these chemical reactions are carried out in the liver, which metabolizes not only drugs but also nearly all of the other foreign chemicals we take into our bodies. Processing by the liver, therefore, is a critical factor not only in drug therapy but also in defending our brains and bodies against the toxic effects of environmental chemicals such as insecticides, herbicides, dyes, certain food preservatives, and a number of other substances.

At approximately three pounds, your liver is the largest organ in your body. It is your primary receiving depot, chemical processing plant, and distribution center for almost everything that enters your body through the walls of your digestive tract. Your liver is also the processing plant for many brain chemicals derived from your food. Glucose, the major fuel for your brain, is produced there, and so are many of the neurotransmitters made from the proteins you eat.

At Rockefeller University Hospital, the oldest free-patient research facility in the nation, healthy volunteers were given diets and drugs to test interactions. Food was meticulously weighed and measured.

Dr. Kappas points out that diet is a major point of direct contact between us and our external environment, yet relatively little attention has been paid to the interaction between food and drugs given for treatment. "Vegetables, for example, contain a variety of chemicals. The effect of these chemicals on our bodies is not fully known. It has been observed, for example, that cruciferous vegetables such as brussels sprouts and cabbage increase the metabolism of certain drugs," he said, "and such an effect could alter the drugs' actions."[4]

Physicians may manipulate people's diets—for example, in cases of obesity, fat-clogged arteries, and diabetes—and yet make no changes in medications, although such changes may be needed. According to Dr. Kappas, many healthy people manipulate diets on their own, particularly for weight loss, without telling their physicians so that medications for other problems may be adjusted.

He said that in Rockefeller University Hospital experiments, protein and carbohydrate intakes in the diet of healthy men were altered to determine the effects on metabolism of two prototype drugs; *antipyrine,* a pain killer that is incompatible with iron and iodine (see pages 54–55), and *theophylline,* which acts as a diuretic, heart stimulant, and smooth-muscle relaxant. Both drugs depend on liver enzymes for processing.

Dr. Anderson, now a professor of preventive medicine at the University of Texas Medical Center, Galveston, recalled how difficult it was to raise the protein in the diet to 40 to 50 percent in the Rockefeller experiments: "The average diet in the United States, which is considered high protein, has about 10 to 14 percent protein. We raised the protein level by giving tuna fish, poultry, meat, and a protein supplement. For the high-carbohydrate diet, we gave them pasta, vegetables, bread, and candy."[5] When the men in the study ate a low-carbohydrate, high-protein diet, it took the subjects an average of 50 percent less time to clear the drugs from their bodies than it did when a high-carbohydrate, low-protein diet was eaten.

High-protein diets can speed up the rate of drug metabolism, as can non-nutrient components of the diet such as flavonoids and indoles, the Rockefeller investigators concluded. (*Flavonoids* are substances derived from plants and perform varying biological activities. They are often used in foods to keep metals from oxidizing and affecting the taste of fats, oils, and salad dressings. *Indoles* are synthetic flavoring agents extracted from coal tar and feces in highly dilute solutions. They are used in raspberry, strawberry, bitters, chocolate, orange, coffee, violet, fruit, nut, and cheese flavorings for beverages, ice cream, ices, candy, baked goods, and gelatin desserts.)

Dr. Kappas said he and Dr. Anderson obtained evidence that in healthy people, alterations in the relative amounts of carbohydrates and proteins in the diet can alter the metabolism of steroid hormones in the liver. Steroids from your sex and adrenal glands greatly affect your brain, behavior, and mood. Dramatic examples, of course, are the symptoms of premenstrual tension caused by sex steroids or the rapid heartbeat and sweating produced by the steroids from the adrenals.

"This finding that diet can alter the processing of steroids by the liver has important implications because it has been clearly established that steroid hormone metabolites (breakdown products) have potent biologic properties of their own and [that] these may differ significantly from those of their parent hormones,"[6] Dr. Kappas says.

Cooking foods at high temperatures can also alter our metabolism when we ingest certain foods, especially if we eat lots of charbroiled meats. Those taking the asthma drug theophylline, for example, should skip the barbecues. Interaction between theophylline and the hydrocarbons from cooking make the medicine 22 percent less effective.

Charcoal broiling, Dr. Kappas says, produces cancer-causing chemicals, some of which are similar to those found in cigarette smoke. It is well known that cigarette smoking accelerates the metabolism of certain drugs and chemicals in the smoker.

Dr. Kappas claims there may be five hundred times more of certain

hydrocarbons in a large charbroiled steak than there are in a pack of
cigarettes, and that carcinogens that accumulate in some shellfish, certain teas, and decaffeinated coffees may considerably exceed the amounts
found in smoke taken into the lungs of cigarette smokers.

Of course, Dr. Kappas is not in favor of cigarette smoking. He is
simply in favor of everyone being more aware that chemicals in foods and
medicines are not innocuous and may have untoward effects on our
bodies and brains because of interactions. (Asked what he has in his own
medicine chest at home, Dr. Kappas would admit to only a jar of shaving
cream, a tube of toothpaste, and a bottle of aspirin. He says he rarely
opens the last.[7])

Dr. Kappas notes that as we grow older, the possibility of untoward
drug effects increases. The usual drug dosages recommended for adults
are based on the assumption that the medication will be inactivated or
removed from our bodies fast enough to prevent an excess from building
up in our blood and tissue. Our livers and kidneys play the major role
in clearing most drugs from our systems. During the passage of time,
these organs become less efficient—even if we are perfectly healthy. Our
brains and hearts are particularly sensitive to drugs in later years. That
means over-the-counter products as well as prescription medications.[8]

Dr. Anderson points out that very few studies have been done to
investigate what happens to foods and drugs together as they are processed by the liver. He intends to carry his studies of food-drug interactions further: "All our studies at Rockefeller were done with normal,
healthy people. I now want to continue the work with patients and with
older people whose livers metabolize drugs and food more slowly. I want
to see whether the slower metabolism by the liver is due to aging or
whether a gradual change in diet over many years may cause the liver
to slow down. We do know that older people don't eat as much protein
in later years as they did when younger."[9]

Included in his new studies will be the effects of certain drugs aimed
at the brain. "We want to study the common tranquilizers and sleeping
pills, the benzodiazepines, as well as the widely used analgesic,
acetaminophen [Tylenol],"[10] says Anderson. The investigation is complicated, he points out, because the liver has not just one enzyme system
but many, and because it is a factory producing numerous products.

The study of the interaction of foods and drugs does not concern just
the liver and its enzymes, however. Foods can slow or impair absorption
of drugs taken by mouth in several ways. Heavy meals, hot meals, and

high-fat meals delay stomach emptying and therefore delay the rate of passage of drugs into the small intestine, where most drugs are absorbed through the very large, crinkly surfaces of the intestinal walls. The longer a drug resides in your stomach due to your having eaten a meal, the more time it has to disintegrate and dissolve in your stomach.

Eating food increases blood flow, which, in turn, can alter absorption and speed of effect. Liquids, for example, may accelerate emptying the stomach, whereas solids can delay it. In some cases, food can inhibit drug absorption by acting as a mechanical barrier between drug molecules and the intestinal wall or by causing digestive juices to flow into the gastrointestinal tract. Thus, the presence of food in the gastrointestinal tract can reduce, delay, or increase drug absorption, or it may have no effect, depending on the composition of the meal and on the chemical ingredients in the drug.[11]

The presence of food in the stomach can affect the way in which some drugs are absorbed. Some drugs are absorbed better with food in the stomach and some are absorbed better when there is no food in the stomach. A delay in absorption of a drug because of food in the stomach may just mean that it takes longer for a drug to do its job. Or it may mean that the drug has been rendered ineffective. The chart on page 126 lists some common examples.

Just as foods can affect the benefits you may derive from medications, medications may sabotage absorption of nutrients from your meals. Numerous drugs have been shown to adversely affect the absorption of nutrients from food. That malabsorption can be *primary* and due to the direct effects of a medication on the workings of the intestines, or the malabsorption can be *secondary* and occur when one nutrient interferes with the absorption, disposition, or metabolism of another.

Two examples of drugs that cause secondary malabsorption are the anticonvulsant phenytoin (Dilantin), which suppresses vitamin D absorption, and oral contraceptives, which can cause poor absorption of the B vitamins, particularly folacin and B_{12}. The lack of folacin then induces malabsorption of other nutrients (see chapter 3).

What effects do combinations of foods and drugs have on our brains? If an adverse interaction occurs and you feel rotten, of course it will influence your ability to function mentally. There are, however, some direct effects on the brain, as in Charlie's and Sandy's cases, described at the beginning of this chapter.

THE EFFECT OF FOOD IN THE STOMACH ON THE ABSORPTION OF CERTAIN DRUGS

IMPROVED ABSORPTION WITH FOOD	DELAYED ABSORPTION WITH FOOD	REDUCED ABSORPTION WITH FOOD
Vitamins	*Antibiotics*	*Antibiotics*
Urinary Antibiotics	Amoxicillin	Penicillin
Nitrofuradantin	Cephalexin	Ampicillin
Antifungals	Sulfa drugs	Tetracycline
Griseofulvin	*Pain Killers*	*Anti-Parkinsonisms*
High Blood Pressure	Aspirin	L-dopa
Medications	Acetaminophen	*Anti-TB's*
Propananol	*Heart Medications*	Rifampicin
Metroprolol	Digoxin	Isonazid
Hydrazaline	*Diuretics*	*Sedatives*
Spironolactone	Furosemide	Phenobarbital
Anticonvulsants	*Supplements*	*Supplements*
Pain Killers	Potassium	Calcium
Propoxyphene	*Tranquilizers*	
(Darvon)	Diazepam (Valium)	
Mefenamic Acid		
(Ponstel)		

DRUGS THAT CAUSE LOW BLOOD SUGAR

An injection of insulin can affect the areas of the brain involved in the sensation of hunger in both diabetics and nondiabetics who haven't eaten for at least six hours. Insulin, by design, causes blood sugar to fall. If it falls too low, then instead of a desire for food, sensations of nausea and weakness may occur.

A sudden drop in blood sugar can cause fainting, coma, and, eventually, death. Whether or not an insulin injection was given and, if it was, by whom, were the unanswered questions in the famous Rhode Island case in which Klaus Von Bulow was accused of giving his millionairess wife Sunny a near-fatal injection of insulin. Since Sonny reportedly suffered from low blood sugar, an injection of insulin could have caused the coma from which she never recovered. This type of low blood sugar problem may also develop when diabetic patients taking blood sugar lowering drugs orally drink alcohol. Alcohol, when swallowed on top of an antidiabetic drug, can cause blood sugar to dip too low and produce such symptoms as weakness, mental confusion, irrational behavior, and loss of consciousness.

But even people without diabetes or a low blood sugar problem can have a drop in blood sugar by combining certain foods, alcohol, and drugs.

ALCOHOL, FOOD, AND DRUGS

Alcohol is absorbed more rapidly from the stomach in the absence of food, and, very often, meals are skipped by drinkers because liquor kills appetite. All else being equal, people who drink on an empty stomach will develop higher blood levels of alcohol than will those who drink during or after eating. For example, the 125-pound person who gets half way to the legal blood-alcohol limit with just two drinks might need four drinks to reach the same level if she drinks within two hours after eating the equivalent of a full meal. People who do not eat (and thus have a low blood sugar) and then have a few cocktails, especially those made with a sweet mix such as gin and tonic, could very easily have an accident if they get behind the wheel of an automobile.[12]

Removal of alcohol from the blood is affected by two major factors—time and a healthy liver—as pointed out before in this chapter. Persons with severe liver disease or those consuming certain drugs may have livers that are inefficient in removing alcohol from the blood. But even a healthy liver can get rid of only about one drink per hour—a twelve-ounce can of beer, a five-ounce glass of wine, or one mixed drink. More than that, especially in a person of small build with an empty stomach, and trouble starts rising in the blood.[13]

Alcohol can affect almost any drug, and a high intake of alcohol with drugs, especially in people who ordinarily do not consume much alcohol, slows the rate of drug metabolism and increases toxicity.

Whether you call it a food or a drug, alcohol dampens the activity of the central nervous system, which means that it can increase the sedative effects of a long list of medicines that also act on the brain. When central nervous system depressant drugs, such as sleeping pills, antihistamines, tranquilizers, and narcotic analgesics, are taken with alcoholic beverages, the result can be loss of consciousness and death. This reportedly was the cause of death in the case of Dorothy Kilgallen, a well-known newspaper columnist in the 1960s who died after ingesting cocktails and then taking a sleeping pill.

The following are some examples of drug-alcohol interactions:

- When combined with the muscle relaxant Valium or any other benzodiazepine, the effect of alcohol on the brain and on coordination is greatly increased in amounts as small as two ounces of alcohol.

- Alcohol and codeine, which are paired in many cough syrup formulations, increase central nervous system impairment. When such medications are in the bloodstream, one drink can have the effect of two or three.

- If an older person takes nitroglycerin under the tongue or by mouth and then drinks alcohol, a severe drop in blood pressure can occur.

- Alcohol taken with certain sulfa drugs can cause flushing, headache, nausea, vomiting, and chest and abdominal pain. *Griseofulvin* (an antifungal medicine) or *tetrachloroethylene* (an antiworm medicine) taken with alcohol can cause flushing, headache, and shortness of breath.

The interactive effects of food, drugs, and alcohol are more obvious than perhaps any other combination, particularly on the brain.

One drug that interacts with alcohol and causes nausea and vomiting is disulfiram (Antabuse). It is, in fact, used medically for that very purpose—to give alcoholics the self-control needed to avoid drinking liquor. They know in advance that if they don't avoid alcohol, they will become nauseous.

Alcohol also has a direct effect on the brain (see pages 145–148), but its effect, especially in the unborn, is increased when protein is low in the diet. The brains of babies born to mothers who drink heavily are not only smaller than brains of babies born to nondrinkers, but also they are prone to disconnections in the corpus callosum, the switchboard between the two halves of the brain.[14]

Alcohol is not the only common player in the food-drug interaction field. Certain popular vegetables can affect your body's use of medications, too.

THE BUTTERFLY AND THE CABBAGE

The butterfly-shaped thyroid gland in your neck is the "governor" of metabolism, the regulator of the rate at which your body consumes oxygen. Thyroid hormone is required for normal growth and development of the brain and of muscles and bones. It indirectly affects the activity of your other glands of internal secretion. Too little thyroid hormone produces a slow metabolic rate and therefore slows down all of your body's chemical processing. For good thyroid function there must be normal pituitary gland function, sufficient iodine intake from food and water, and normal manufacture and release of thyroid hormone by the gland. In addition to lack of iodine in the diet, too little thyroid hormone can be due to diseases of the brain areas that regulate the thyroid gland or destruction of thyroid tissue by inflammation. Among the symptoms of a low thyroid output are slow speech, weight gain, general apathy and fatigue, emotional changes easily confused with depression or senility, and, in the extreme, coma. Treatment for the condition consists of taking supplemental thyroid hormone, which should be taken before eating in the morning. If you are taking thyroid medication, it would be best to avoid excessive intake of kale, cabbage, carrots, peas, cauliflower, spinach, turnips, rutabagas, soybean products, peaches, beans, and brussels sprouts. All of these vegetables contain substances that can inhibit the activity of the thyroid hormone and interfere with thyroid therapy.[15]

And while some foods, like the vegetables above, can interfere with medication, some medications can deplete nutrient absorption. Chronic ingestion of aspirin, for example, can deplete the body's store of B vitamins, particularly folic acid. Deficiencies of the B vitamins have been found to lead to pseudosenility among some elderly patients.[16] Aspirin and alcohol taken together can increase the risk of stomach irritation and internal bleeding. Diabetic patients who are taking tablets to lower their blood sugar may experience serious decreases in their blood sugar if they also take aspirin.

ANTIDEPRESSANTS AND FOOD INTERACTIONS

As pointed out before, if you are taking an antidepressant medication, avoid alcohol. You should also avoid large amounts of alkaline foods, because they will cause your urine to become alkaline. Alkaline urine prolongs the effect of these drugs in the body. Diet alone is not likely to cause alkaline urine unless you frequently ingest alkaline foods or are a vegetarian or a chronic antacid taker. If you are on antidepressants, it would be prudent to use the following alkaline foods sparingly:

Milk	Coconuts
Buttermilk	All vegetables except corn and lentils
Almonds	All fruits except cranberries, plums, and prunes
Chestnuts	

The list of known food-drug interactions is growing longer as scientists gather more information. For example, a chelating agent (chelation removes metals) such as D-penicillamine (used in the treatment of certain kidney problems, heavy metal poisonings, and rheumatoid arthritis) may produce a loss of taste. Caffeine is in many analgesics, headache pills, antihistamines, and pep pills. Caffeine impairs the absorption of iron. Coffee and tea, as well as drugs containing caffeine, may affect the active ingredients of major tranquilizers, thereby weakening the benefits of these medications.

The chart on the following pages shows some food-drug interactions.

As far as helping to prevent untoward food-drug interactions in your life, do the following:

- Remember that foods as well as drugs are composed of chemicals.

- Recognize that over-the-counter medications, including vitamins, are drugs and may interact with foods.

- Before you take any medication, ask both your physician and your pharmacist about potential food-drug interactions and whether you should take the medicine with meals or between meals, and read the package inserts carefully.

- Avoid any alcoholic beverages when taking medications.

- Ask yourself if you really need the aid of a medication or whether a walk, a hot bath, or a rest will do just as well. The fewer drug-food combinations you ingest, the lower your chances of having a bad reaction.

WHEN TAKING THESE DRUGS	IT'S BEST TO AVOID THESE FOODS	ADVERSE EFFECTS
Anticonvulsants		
Carbamazepine (Tegretol)	Alcohol	Sodium loss, water retention, loss of appetite, vomiting, weakness, seizures, constipation, rash, and pulmonary dysfunction
Phenobarbital	Milk, cream, coconuts, almonds, chestnuts, and buttermilk	Rash, drowsiness
	Alcohol	Vitamin B_{12}, B_6, D, and K deficiencies
Phenytoin (Dilantin)	Alcohol	Reduces effect of and depletes vitamins D, K, and folic Acid
Primidone (Mysoline)	Alcohol	Reduces effect of vitamins D, K, and folic acid
Analgesics		
Acetaminophen	Alcohol; vitamin C over 500 milligrams per day	Gastrointestinal upset, damage to kidneys, and inability to regulate body fluids
Sodium bicarbonate (Alka-Seltzer)	Salty foods, excess milk and dairy products, acid foods such as fruit juices, caffeine	Nutrient deficiencies, salt retention (which elevates blood pressure)
Aspirin (acetylsalicylic acid)	Alcohol	Depletes vitamins B_1, K, C, and folic acid Can cause bleeding, irritated stomach
Decadron	Salty foods; fatty foods	Heart failure due to potassium loss Bone pain due to calcium loss, water retention, disturbed sugar metabolism, loss of vitamins B_6, C, and zinc

TABLE—*Continued*

WHEN TAKING THESE DRUGS	IT'S BEST TO AVOID THESE FOODS	ADVERSE EFFECTS
Heart Medication		
Quinidine	Alkaline foods such as buttermilk, coconut, and some vegetables	Builds up to toxic levels and can affect heart rhythms
High Blood Pressure Drugs		
Chlorothiazide (Hydrochlorthiazide; Hydrodiuril)	Alcohol	Loss of body water
Reserpine	Foods containing tyramine: liver, raisins, avocados, yeast, MSG, bananas, licorice, salty foods, and alcohol	Gastrointestinal upset, worsens ulcers, and water retention

⧫ 8 ⧫

Have You Eaten Any Neurotoxins Lately?

---

*H*arry, *an engineer in his early thirties, had very severe headaches that would last up to three days. As time passed, they became increasingly frequent and severe, and he seemed to be constantly irritable. Harry went to a kaleidoscope of doctors and each time received a prescription for another pain killer. Because his stomach bothered him, he kept taking mints and antacids.* [1]

In the meantime, his small daughter, Laura, also had a very low tolerance for frustration. She was easily distracted, although she was not physically hyperactive.

Jane, the wife and mother in this family, taught art at a local grammar and junior high school. She felt she could not return to her job after Laura was born because she found it difficult to cope with the child's behavior. Jane talked to other mothers about her problem, and one of them suggested she buy a book that described a diet free of artificial colorings and flavorings and natural salicylates. Jane bought the book and started purchasing food and cooking meals according to the instructions.

Not only did Laura's behavior problems disappear, but so did Harry's headaches subside. Today, Laura is a seventeen-year-old honor student in high school. Harry is headache-free, and Jane Hersey is executive director of the Feingold Association of the United States. [2]

The organization and the diet are based on the work of the late Dr. Benjamin Feingold, who was chief of allergy at Kaiser Permanente Medical Center in San Francisco. In 1973, Dr. Feingold presented a paper at a meeting of the American Medical Association purporting that adverse reactions to artificial food additives and natural salicylates were

133

manifested as hyperactivity in some children. He said the adverse reactions did not involve the immune system but instead were due to druglike sensitivities.

Dr. Feingold later wrote a best seller, *Why Your Child Is Hyperactive* (Random House, 1975). Today, according to Jane Hersey, there are ten thousand members of the Feingold organization and an estimated two hundred thousand families who follow the regimen. Many scientists, however, believe artificial food additives and natural salicylates are harmless, and argue that the diet and behavioral changes in families like the Hersheys are merely coincidental.

The Feingold Association* lists the following symptoms as being possibly related to sensitivity to synthetic additives or salicylates:

Symptoms
Marked hyperactivity and fidgetiness
Excitability, impulsivity
Poor sleep habits
Short attention span
Clumsiness
Poor hand-eye coordination
Difficulty with buttoning, writing, drawing, and speech
Trouble with comprehension and memory

Substances on Feingold "Don't Eat" List
Synthetic (artificial) colors
Synthetic (artificial) flavors
Preservatives:
  BHA (butylated hydroxyanisole),
  BHT (butylated hydroxytoluene),
  TBHQ (monotertiary butylhydroxylquinone)
Natural Salicylates
  Almonds
  Apples (also cider and cider vinegar)
  Apricots
  All berries
  Cherries
  Cloves

*The Feingold Association of the United States is located at P.O. Box 6550, Alexandria, Va. 22306

Coffee
Cucumbers and pickles
Currants
Grapes and raisins
   (also wine and wine vinegar)
Green peppers
   (also chilies)
Nectarines
Oranges
Peaches
Plums and prunes
Tangerines
Tea
Tomatoes
Oil of wintergreen

Dr. Bernard Weiss of the radiation biology and biophysics department at the University of Rochester School of Medicine and colleagues from the Kaiser Foundation Research Institute and the University of California did one of the first tightly controlled tests of the Feingold Diet and its effects on hyperactivity in children.[3] Twenty-two youngsters were maintained on a diet that excluded artificial flavorings and colorings and then were intermittently given a blend of seven artificial colors in a double-blind trial. That is, the investigators, the children, and the children's parents and teachers did not know when the artificial colors were given. The colors were in soft drinks identical to soft drinks that had inert substances.

Of the twenty-two youngsters, one responded mildly to the challenge and another responded dramatically. The latter, a thirty-four-month-old girl, showed a significant increase in agitation. Dr. Weiss and his colleagues concluded that certain youngsters *are* sensitive to artificial additives and that the reason other studies had been negative was because insufficient amounts of the chemicals due to deficiencies in experimental analysis.

Because of the controversy over diet and hyperactivity, the National Institutes of Health held a consensus development conference on "Defined Diets and Hyperactivity" in January 1982. A vocal contingent of physicians and families of hyperactive children contended that "defined diets" that are free of artificial colors, flavors, and preservatives are an effective treatment for childhood hyperactivity. An equally vocal contingent of medical researchers asserted that the diets' effects, if any, should be ascribed to faith healing.

Walking a tightrope between seeming to endorse the defined diets and condemning them outright as unproved in controlled studies, the consensus panel concluded that parents and physicians who believe in the diets may want to give them a try. But the panel made it clear that there is no firm evidence.

The controversy continues. In 1985, an article was published in the British medical journal *Lancet* about the results of a well-controlled study. Seventy-six hyperactive children were given a diet consisting typically of two meats (such as lamb and chicken), two carbohydrates (such as potatoes and rice), two fruits, vegetables, water, calcium, and vitamins for the first four weeks. Those whose behavior was improved on the simple diet were then given fruit juices with artificial colorings and the preservative benzoic acid. If the symptoms returned, they were asked to participate in a double-blind study in which neither researchers nor subjects knew when the suspect chemicals were administered. The results were that, on the restricted diet, sixty-two children improved and a normal range of behavior was achieved in twenty-one of the children. Other symptoms such as headaches, abdominal pains, and tantrums also were relieved. Twenty-eight of the children who improved in the first weeks of the diet had their symptoms return or made worse when they were again given the additives, but not when they were given a placebo. In addition, one food dye, Yellow no. 5, and a preservative, sodium benzoate, produced the greatest adverse reactions in the children.

The University of Rochester's Dr. Weiss points out that Yellow no. 5 is banned in a number of European countries because it causes reactions in people who are sensitive to aspirin. He said there are a lot of questions about Yellow no. 6 and Red no. 40 because there are relatively high levels of these additives in food.

FD & C Red no. 40 is the newest and last general-purpose red coloring used in American foods. Yellow no. 6 is a coal tar dye used in carbonated beverages, gelatin desserts, candy, and other confections.

One of the most suspect food additives, as far as the brain is concerned, however, is FD & C Red no. 3 *(erythrosine)*. A coal tar derivative, it is used in canned fruit cocktail, fruit and cherry pie mix (up to .01 percent), maraschino cherries, gelatin desserts, ice cream, sherbet, candy, confectionery products, bakery products, cereal, and pudding. When erythrosine was applied to isolated nerves in the muscles of frogs, it increased the release of the neurotransmitter acetylcholine. The University of Maryland investigators who performed this study said the results suggested that erythrosine might prove useful as a tool for studying the process of transmitter release but that its use as a food additive should be reexamined. George J. Augustine, Jr., and Herbert Levitan of the zoology department at the University of Maryland said:

> Our observation that a widely used food coloring agent, such as erythrosine, could dramatically and irreversibly alter synaptic transmission [messages across the gap between nerves] at low doses is consistent with previous studies suggesting that this and other food additives can alter behavior. While it may be tempting to use these in vitro findings to support claims that these substances would cause behavioral changes when ingested by laboratory animals or humans, such conclusions are premature until it can be determined whether this and other additives have access to the central nervous system. It is not yet known how much of the ingested dye—it was estimated in 1968 that the maximum daily ingestion was 2 milligrams per person—is free in the blood or how readily it crosses the blood brain barrier.[5]

Jane Hersey of the Feingold Association says that the argument today is not over *if* the Feingold Diet (which excludes artificial colorings and flavorings) works, but rather over *why* it works and how many children can benefit.

Chemicals that we eat and drink intentionally or unintentionally may adversely affect our brains and nerves, and yet only now are regulatory agencies beginning to develop regulations and test for them. The task is formidable, since there are more than 70,000 chemicals in use and about 615 added to the marketplace each year. By 1990, it is expected that there will be 363 million pounds of food additives added each year to processed meat alone.[6]

Charles Vorhees, Ph.D., associate professor of pediatrics and developmental biology at the Institute for Developmental Research, Children's Hospital Research Foundation, and the University of Cincinnati, points out: "The fact that food can produce adverse effects on behavior has long been known but efforts to systematically evaluate foods and other chemicals for such effects are a more recent pursuit."[7] The fields that have evolved to assess these effects have come to be termed:

Behavioral toxicology: The study of chemical effects on mature organisms.

Behavioral teratology: The part of behavioral toxicology that focuses on the unborn and the newborn and the consequences for later life of exposure during these key periods of brain development. The young organism is more susceptible to many chemicals and the aftermath of exposure is more likely to be permanent in children than in adults.[8]

George Wagner, Ph.D., of Rutgers University studies neurotoxins. He believes that the brains of older people may be more vulnerable to certain chemicals, particularly in the areas involving dopamine, the neurotransmitter involved in movement. He says that it is possible that an acute effect can cause damage, but that damage may only become evident later when the enzymes in the aging brain change or when there is an accumulation of exposures that produce increasingly large lesions over the years.[9]

Dr. Vorhees, Dr. Wagner, and other neurotoxicologists agree that while other areas of the body may be vulnerable in both children and adults, the brain may be said to be the organ most sensitive to damage. Behavioral symptoms, they say, can be a more sensitive index of developmental injury than visible physical birth defects.

The relatively young discipline of behavioral toxicology came into existence in 1975, when Dr. Weiss and his colleague, Dr. V. G. Laties, pointed out that adverse effects of environmental agents need not be limited to tissue pathology. Brain function deficits can be equally disabling, and the environment exposes us to many agents that act on the nervous system. Heavy metals such as lead and mercury, fuels and solvents such as methanol and carbon disulfide, and pesticides are among such chemicals.

The University of Rochester's Dr. Weiss, however, expressed frustration at trying to test neurotoxicity in foods.[10] He said the food industry has had a massive publicity campaign against the Feingold Diet, for example, and even when the researchers the industry hired to refute the premise came up with some positive findings, only the negative results were publicized.

The University of Rochester professor says there is little funding to study neurotoxins in foods even though there is a great need to do so.

An international research team found strong evidence that a poisonous substance in a plant eaten widely on Guam during World War II was the cause of the devastating brain and nerve disease that appeared years afterward among natives of that Pacific island.[11] An amino acid, *beta methylamino-L-alanine,* was implicated in the Guam disorder. The scientists fed monkeys moderate amounts of the chemical and found that the animals developed severe nerve disorders. The severity of the disease and the time it took for symptoms to develop depended on the amount the animals ate.

The chemical is found in a type of cycad seed that the Guam natives ate during World War II when food was scarce. The greatest number of cases of nerve and brain damage showed up about ten years later.

Dr. Peter Spencer, a leader of the research team and director of the Institute of Neurotoxicology at the Albert Einstein College of Medicine, observed that the evidence warrants a search for comparable environmental factors in several diseases, including Alzheimer's, that destroy the brain and nervous system. He said the role of early exposure to neurotoxic substances in such diseases should be investigated.[12]

There are scientists who now believe that slow-acting neurotoxins or constant ingestion of minute amounts of neurotoxins may cause cognitive and behavior problems in both young and old. One of the most controversial areas targeted involves those chemicals intentionally or unintentionally added to our food supply.

Rochester's Dr. Weiss says that behavioral toxicity is not yet a component of standard food additive safety testing, but that the absence of behavioral criteria from food additive test protocols is beginning to seem curious: "The FDA is interested in contamination of food and in testing for cancer-causing agents but it doesn't make sense not to test for neurotoxins. There are many more instances of damage to the nervous system from chemicals than there are of cancers."[13]

LEAD IN THE HEAD

One neurotoxin that has been well studied but that is still with us, despite regulations and massive efforts to get rid of it, is lead. According to the American Academy of Pediatrics, exposure to lead is widespread and causes serious impairments to children at relatively low levels of exposure—the effects of which are largely irreversible.[14]

Lead can cause mental deficiency is children. The main source of chronic lead poisoning was and still is believed to be paint. The use of lead in paint has been banned in the interior of buildings but not in the exterior products. Paint chips can float in the air and be ingested and inhaled by children. Lead can also contaminate acidic foods and beverages (fruits, fruit juices, cola drinks, tomatoes, tomato juice, wine, and cider) by storage in improperly lead-glazed ceramic ware. Commercial canning can also create problems. Freshly opened cans of grapefruit juice and orange juice have lead concentrations that exceed the Environmental Protection Agency (EPA) standard for drinking water, which is 0.05 micrograms per milliliter, says Dennis Bourcier of East Carolina University, Greenville.[15] Lead-soldered cans account for about 14 percent of total human lead ingestion, he adds. Though this solder makes good can seals, children are sensitive to lead and canned juices reach critical lead levels of five times the EPA standard within five days after opening. Juices should be put in nonmetallic containers as soon as they are opened.[16]

ALUMINUM AND ALZHEIMER'S

Is there a connection between aluminum, the third most abundant element on earth, and Alzheimer's, the devastating brain-degenerating disease that affects 2.5 million of middle-aged and older Americans?

Alzheimer's disease was first described in 1906 when Alois Alzheimer, M.D., a German physician, told his colleagues of a fifty-one-year-old woman who had severe atrophy of the brain and an unusual clumping and distortion of fibers in the nerve cells of the cerebral cortex, or outer layer of the brain. The patient's problems began with memory loss and disorientation, progressed to depression and hallucination, and eventually resulted in severe dementia and death.

Dr. Alzheimer did not know what caused the tangles and no one has come up with a proven answer as yet. The National Institutes of Health scientists list three risk factors: family history of the disorder, head trauma, and environmental toxins, particularly aluminum.[17]

The aluminum-intoxication hypothesis got its start when some scientists found brain changes similar to those of Alzheimer's disease in animals that had been injected with aluminum. Other researchers found an excess accumulation of aluminum within the neurofibrillary tangles in the brains of Alzheimer's patients.

Aluminum has also been implicated in dialysis dementia, a frequent side effect of long-term kidney dialysis. However, the brain changes in dialysis patients are not the same as those in Alzheimer's patients. Dr. Weiss says the case against aluminum is not proven, except in dialysis, in which there is a break down of the blood-brain barrier and aluminum can get in. The connection between aluminum and Alzheimer's is hotly debated among researchers working in the field.

You ingest aluminum primarily through foods and drugs, such as antacids and buffered aspirin, although small amounts can come from foods and beverages you store in aluminum cans or cook in aluminum utensils. (The aluminum manufacturers suggest that the questions about aluminum cookware were raised by competitors promoting other types of utensils.)[18] But can aluminum leave your intestines and penetrate the blood-brain barrier?

Dr. Daniel P. Perl, director of neuropathology at the Mount Sinai Medical Center in New York, and an associate, Paul F. Good, reported in the British medical journal *Lancet* that experiments with rabbits showed that aluminum inhaled through the nose can penetrate the brain through the olfactory nerves.[19]

Dr. Perl described various forms of nasal exposure to aluminum, including household substances containing significant amounts of that metal such as baking powder, antiperspirants, buffering compounds, and dust. There were no nerve tangles in Dr. Perl's rabbits, but he is now testing small amounts of aluminum over prolonged periods of time to see if the chronic route is what causes the changes in the brain. He feels the direct route through the nose may be how aluminum gets into the brain, since the intestines and the blood-brain barrier protect the brain from aluminum.

Scientists at the National Institutes of Health, using sophisticated computer-driven electron beam X-ray microprobes, discovered a surprising correlation between certain elements and nerve-damaged brains. They found silicon, which is derived from silica and used as an anticaking agent in foods; calcium, the mineral needed for strong bones and teeth; and aluminum in nerve tangles in certain areas of the brains of victims with the degenerating nerve disorder Lou Gehrig's disease (amyotrophic lateral sclerosis) and in those with Parkinsonism with dementia.[20]

A similar mechanism may be involved in Alzheimer's disease, as silicon and aluminum have been found in nerve tangles in Alzheimer's victims' brains. Silicon, like aluminum, may interfere with the transmission of nerve messages. FDA officials, however, maintain that no direct causative effect between aluminum and Alzheimer's disease has been shown to date.[21]

Nevertheless, if you want to cut down your ingestion of aluminum, you can follow these simple precautions:

• Avoid digestion tablets containing aluminum

• Avoid underarm deodorant sprays containing aluminum (sprays are easily inhaled)

• Avoid aluminum saucepans when cooking acidic foods

• Avoid processed foods with aluminum food additives listed on the label (see below)

ALUMINUM FOOD ADDITIVES

Alum: Used in food packaging and to harden gelatin.

Aluminum ammonium sulfate: Used to purify drinking water; in baking powder; as a buffering and neutralizing agent in milling and in the cereal industry.

Aluminum calcium sulfate: Anticaking agent used in table salt and vanilla powder.

Aluminum hydroxide: An alkali used as a leavening agent in baked goods.

Aluminum nicotinate: Used as a source of niacin in special diet foods.

Aluminum oleate: Used in food packaging.

Aluminum palmitate: Used in packaging.

Aluminum phosphide: Used to fumigate processed foods.

Aluminum potassium sulfate (potash alum; potassium alum): Used as a firming agent in sugar processing and as a carrier for bleaching agent. It is used in the production of sweet and dill pickles, cereal, flours, bleached flours, and cheese.

Aluminum sodium sulfate: A firming agent and carrier for bleaching agents.

Aluminum stearate: Used in chewing gum bases and as a defoaming agent in beet sugar and yeast processing.

Aluminum sulfate (cake alum; pat- *ent alum):* A firming agent used in processing sweet and dill pickles and as a modifier for food starch.

Sodium silico aluminate: An anticaking agent used in table salt (up to 2 percent), in dried egg yolks (up to 2 percent), in sugar (up to 1 percent), and in baking powder (up to 5 percent).

Neurotoxins are not necessarily chemicals that are hidden in our food or drink or that are put there against our will. They may be substances that we take by choice because they make us feel better or because we prefer the taste or look when they are in a dish or glass.

THE HANGOVER BRAIN

Two of the most common psychoactive substances ingested—alcohol and caffeine—can have an adverse effect on nerves.

If you have ever had a hangover or staggered around after one too many cocktails, your brain has experienced the obvious neurotoxicity of alcohol. What actually happens when you down that glass of beer or wine or shot of liquor?

Alcohol speeds through your body. It doesn't have to be digested. It can be absorbed into your blood stream directly from your stomach wall and small intestine. Its effects always are determined by the amount in your blood. When you finish an average drink—wine, beer, or a cocktail—the alcohol is carried by your bloodstream to every cell in your body.

The most visible damage is to your central nervous system. If you are moderately intoxicated, you may experience a "loosening of the tongue" and a lowering of your inhibitions, because the part of your brain that controls your reason and judgment is affected first. As the level of alcohol in your blood rises, the drug becomes a depressant, causing your mood to change and your sexual performance, especially if you are male, to be impaired. Alcohol then affects your coordination, depth perception, and reflex actions. Alcohol can dilate the blood vessels in your brain and put you into the characteristic morning-after-the-night-before state.

This "hangover" can muddle your thinking and coordination long after the headache and malaise are not obvious. Stanford University researchers reported in the *American Journal of Psychiatry* on alcohol-impaired pilots' cockpit performances fourteen hours after the flyers had their last drink. The study showed that a hangover can harm a pilot's cockpit performance even when alcohol is no longer detectable in his bloodstream. Furthermore, the pilot may not be aware of the impairment.[22]

Dr. John Brick, laboratory director of the Alcohol Behavior Research Laboratory at Rutgers University, said there are several possible explanations for alcohol affecting performance, as in the case of the pilots, after the substance has disappeared from the blood. The most likely explanation involve changes in the central nervous system caused by intoxication. Nerve signals may not come back to their original states immediately upon the removal of alcohol but instead may take some time to readjust.

This newly recognized time lag for the neurological effects of alcohol to dissipate has led the Federal Aviation Commission to reevaluate the eight-hour requirement for pilot alcohol abstinence before flights.[23]

This long delay in getting alcohol out of the system should not be that surprising. It has long been known that alcohol withdrawal symptoms usually occur between twenty-five and forty-eight hours after the last drink and that delirium tremens occur three or four days later. Such a delay often complicates care.[24]

The d.t.'s are associated with chronic drinking. But what about people who just overdo it occasionally? In most states, you are considered legally drunk when one of every thousand parts of your blood (0.1 percent) is composed of pure alcohol. In some people this can occur when any more than two drinks are ingested within an hour. At 0.2 percent alcohol (5 or more drinks in a short time) the midbrain is affected and you stagger, perhaps dropping off to sleep. At 0.3 percent you are very drunk and in a confused stupor. At 0.4 percent you might become comatose and require hospitalization.

If you raise your blood levels to over 0.3 percent alcohol, the activity of your lungs, heart, breathing, and circulation are greatly depressed. The expression "dead drunk" comes from the fact that alcohol has the potential to completely paralyze breathing and cause death. This tragedy has happened a number of times during fraternity pledging when candidates were forced to drink a lot of alcohol in a short period of time.

More commonly, alcohol takes a longer time to do its damage. The link between heavy alcohol consumption and loss of gray matter has long been suspected but now has been precisely measured. Heavy drinking shrinks the brain, according to a report in the *British Medical Journal.* [25] The brains of the alcoholics studied weighed an average 105 grams less than those of teetotalers or moderate drinkers. The brains of forty-four people who died at an average age of fifty-eight years were examined. Half had been drinking heavily for at least thirty or forty years and their brains weighed an average of 1,315 grams. The other half, who were either teetotalers or who drank well within the safety limits of alcohol intake, had brains weighing 1,420 grams.

In 1981, Charles J. Golden and his colleagues at the University of Nebraska Medical Center reported that computerized X-rays, or CAT scans, of eleven chronic alcoholics averaging just over twenty-nine years of age revealed reductions in density in their left hemispheres but not in their right. These results suggest that the logical-thinking left hemisphere is more sensitive than the right hemisphere to the effect of alcohol and that significant brain changes can occur at a fairly early age among alcoholics. [26]

ALCOHOL AND STROKE

Alcohol abuse is the nation's number one health problem in terms of costs to the economy. About $117 billion a year are spent, most of it in lost productivity. The direct treatment costs for alcoholism amount to about $13.5 billion a year. [27]

More than 10.6 million people are alcoholics and an additional 7.3 million either are alcohol abusers or have experienced negative consequences of alcohol use such as arrest or involvement in an automobile accident. In addition, an estimated 4.6 million young people aged fourteen to seventeen are problem drinkers. An estimated one-third to one-half of all unintentionally and intentionally injured adult Americans involved in accidents, crimes, and suicides have been drinking alcohol. [28]

Alcohol has long been considered a pernicious drug that increases the risk of liver, heart, and lung disease, as well as the risk of involvement in a serious automobile accident. Now stroke can be added to that list, according to researchers from the National Heart, Lung and Blood Institute. Although alcohol consumption has been cited as a risk factor for stroke, its role was thought to be tied to high blood pressure, since alcohol consumption has been documented to increase blood pressure. A study from the Honolulu Heart Program, however, found that alcohol intake is a factor independent of hypertension for increasing the risk of stroke.[29] The study followed more than eight thousand men over twelve years to ascertain the variables associated with the subjects who developed various forms of cerebral vascular accidents. Careful follow-up of all subjects demonstrated that 190 of the original sample experienced a brain hemorrhage, 90 had a blood clot in the brain, and 24 had a stroke of unknown cause.

Similar findings were reported by a London group that studied alcohol consumption among 230 twenty- to seventy-year-old patients with stroke. Among men, the relative risk of stroke, adjusted for high blood pressure, cigarette smoking, and medication, was lower in light drinkers (those consuming 10 to 90 grams of alcohol weekly) than in nondrinkers, but was four times higher in heavy drinkers (those consuming 300 grams of alcohol weekly) than in nondrinkers. This led the Londoners to conclude that heavy alcohol consumption is an important and underrecognized independent risk factor for stroke in men. Their data was not adequate to settle the issue for women.[30]

Researchers report that heavy drinkers of alcohol differ from the general population in several respects. Poor nutrition may be a confounding factor as well as an inherited tendency toward alcohol use. Both of these variables may predispose individuals to a brain hemorrhage, but no one is yet sure why.[31]

People who switch from hard liquor to wine or beer in an effort to protect their brains and bodies from alcohol toxicity aren't helping themselves, says psychiatrist William Hazle, the medical director of the Stanford Alcohol and Drug Treatment Center in Palo Alto, California; "Alcohol is alcohol, and it offers the same potential for addiction in whatever form it's consumed. For example, a standard twelve-ounce bottle or can of beer, a four-ounce glass of wine, or a shot of liquor all provide the same alcohol content."[32]

How much alcohol is too much?

A drink or two can raise your spirits and make you friendlier and more relaxed. Even some research has shown that. But many people can't stop at two drinks, and it may be the inborn way they send messages between their brain cells rather than circumstances that keeps them drinking.

At the National Institutes of Health's Clinic Research Center, 150 participating outpatient alcoholics are receiving a chemical that is converted in the brain to dopamine. Others will receive one that is converted to serotonin. These two neurotransmitters are found in decreased levels in the brains of some alcoholics. Researchers hope that by increasing either serotonin or dopamine, the craving for alcohol may be reduced in alcoholics.[33]

Because males seem to be statistically at greater risk for inheriting alcoholism than females, researchers are also examining the Y chromosome as a source for biological and genetic factors that contribute to alcohol-related problems in males. Studies suggest that a biological relationship may exist among alcoholics, a factor encoded on the Y chromosome and the metabolism of serotonin. In animal studies, rats with low brain serotonin levels have shown a genetic preference for alcohol over water. There is evidence that the gene for this trait may be present on the Y chromosome in humans.

In fact, several lines of evidence converge to suggest that the Y chromosome could be involved in alcoholism and other disorders marked by impulsiveness in males, and that part of the mechanism of alcoholism may be a reduction of serotonin activity in the brain.

Dr. Daniel Goldman, the principal investigator in the National Institutes of Health genetics study, says that when alcohol contacts nerve cell membranes, which are composed of proteins and fatty substances called lipids, it makes the normally viscous membranes more fluid. These altered membranes may cause faulty nerve signal transmission, leading to abnormal brain functioning and scrambled brain messages. Such alcohol-related nerve cell changes may even alter the individual's tolerance to alcohol and perhaps lead to physical dependence and other brain and drinking problems.[34]

Meanwhile, researchers at the laboratory of the National Institutes of Health's Clinical Biochemistry and Pharmacology section are conducting research on twenty normal nonalcoholic men and women to help answer that fundamental question: why does alcohol affect men and women differently? It is known that the blood concentration of alcohol is higher in women than in men after consuming the same size drink. There is speculation that this is a result of the smaller size of women and the smaller amount of water per kilogram of body weight in women. However, this could also be the result of differences in the speed with which the alcohol is eliminated from the body.[35]

Many of the new studies are highlighting brain chemistry as well as life experiences as a factor in alcohol abuse. For example, Conrad M. Swartz, Ph.D., M.D., of the University of Chicago Medical School, reported in 1986 that children and grandchildren of alcoholics who had been adopted at birth and raised by others release much less of the stress neurotransmitter epinephrine in response to mental stress or alcohol than do adopted children who did not have alcoholic biological relatives.[36] The effects of alcohol consumption might be perceived as similar to a state of stress, because both are accompanied by an elevated release of neurotransmitters involved in emotion.

"Our observation that the tendency to alcoholism is associated with less epinephrine release agrees with others findings that in stressful circumstances people with more psychopathic traits release less epinephrine,"[37] wrote Dr. Swartz. He said the Chicago study results also suggest that family alcoholism is associated with a lack of response to the stimulant effects of alcohol rather than to its sedative effects.

A recent study by researchers at Purdue University adds further evidence to this line of thought. The Indiana investigators found that rats put under stress did not drink available alcohol while under stress but only after the stress had stopped.

If the rats' drinking behavior could be equated with humans', it may be that most alcoholics start drinking not when they are under stress but rather when they go home at night and the stress is gone. Then they start drinking because they may be suffering a "withdrawal" from stress.[38]

CAFFEINE "NERVES"

Americans consume about a third of the world's coffee beans. Caffeine is a potent stimulant that acts on the central nervous system and is the most widely used psychoactive substance.

Caffeine is thought to produce its effect by blocking the action of a brain chemical known as *adenosine,* a self-made sedative. Clinical investigators have found that many people with panic attacks avoid caffeine after noticing that it causes attacks.[39]

The effect caffeine has on the brain's neurotransmitters is probably why even moderate amounts of caffeine can trigger and magnify phobias and panic attacks in the estimated two- to six-million Americans afflicted with these disorders. Dr. Thomas Uhde of the National Institute of Mental Health (NIMH) studies panic disorders and reports that people who suffer from these attacks were given caffeine—about four cups' worth of coffee—and then their blood was tested. The NIMH researchers found that the panickers experienced a sharp rise in blood levels of the brain hormone *cortisol* and lactate, a substance known to produce panic attacks. The normal participants who served as comparisons in the tests had no rise in these substances after ingestion of caffeine. Because of the association between caffeine and panic attacks, Dr. Uhde said, some 60 percent of people with disorders will stop drinking coffee before they see a doctor or therapist because they have discovered its exacerbating effect on their illness.[40]

W. Leigh Thompson, M.D., Ph.D., co-director of clinical pharmacology and critical care medicine at Case Western Reserve University, say the effects of caffeine on your brain have a lot to do with whether or not you regularly consume it. If you normally don't drink it, you will feel stimulated after drinking one cup of coffee or tea. You may undergo a slight increase in blood pressure, your kidneys will be stimulated to produce more urine, your body's smooth muscles will be relaxed, and, most noticeably, you will feel awake and alert. If, however, you habitually consume either beverage, you will probably get little caffeine effect. If you ingest about 400 to 500 milligrams (4 to 5 cups) of caffeine a day and show no effects from this large intake, you may have become physically dependent on caffeine. This is due to tolerance: your body's becoming accustomed to a substance.[41]

Since there is such a wide variation in caffeine sensitivity among individuals, caffeine may or may not affect your ability to sleep. Israeli researchers examined rates of clearance of caffeine from plasma in caffeine-sensitive individuals and found them to be an average of some 30 percent lower than in control subjects. Caffeine-sensitive individuals also drank less than average amounts of coffee.[42] Whether differences in rates of clearance are inherited, the product of differential exposure to caffeine, or both, remains to be explored.

Vanderbilt University School of Medicine researchers in Nashville, Tennessee, reported that upon consumption of caffeine thirty to sixty minutes before sleep, some individuals showed delayed sleep onset, a decrease in total sleep time, and reduced subjective estimation of the quality of sleep. However, the researchers noted that tolerance to the effects of caffeine on sleep also occurs. More non-coffee drinkers reported an increase in delayed sleep onset than did habitual heavy coffee drinkers, and non-drinkers showed a greater decrease in sleep quality after coffee consumption.[43] Therefore, if you find that caffeine affects your ability to sleep, you should avoid caffeine for at least five hours before bedtime.

If you decide that you are ingesting too much caffeine daily, don't stop all at once. You can become drowsy, depressed, and develop a headache due to sudden withdrawal. In fact, an article in the *New York State Journal of Medicine* by a physician and a rabbi reported the High Holy Day headaches that some religious patients suffered on Yom Kippur, the Day of Atonement, when a twenty-five-hour fast is customary. Those heavy coffee drinkers in the congregation reported that caffeine withdrawal headaches began about twelve to sixteen hours after their last dose of caffeine. Therefore, if you decide to cut down your caffeine intake, do it gradually over a week or two.[44]

Here's a chart to help you control your caffeine intake:

HIGH-CAFFEINE PRODUCTS

PRODUCT	CAFFEINE CONTENT
Coffee, caffeinated (six-ounce cup)	about 75 to 125 milligrams
Coffee, decaffeinated (six-ounce cup)	about 3 to 5 milligrams
Tea (six-ounce cup)	30 to 65 milligrams
Cocoa (six-ounce cup)	5 milligrams
Bittersweet chocolate (one-ounce piece)	35 milligrams
Soft drinks (twelve-ounce glass)	
Cola	up to 70 milligrams
Seven-up, Sprite	0 milligrams
Over-the-counter drugs, such as antihistamines to fight drowsiness, weight-loss drugs, and stay-awake pills	up to 200 milligrams
Prescription drugs, such as the pain-killers Darvon and Cafergot	32 to 100 milligrams

HOW SWEET IT REALLY IS?

Aspartame is a nutritive sweetener produced commercially from two amino acids, L-phenylalanine and L-aspartic acid. Discovered during a routine screening of drugs for the treatment of ulcers, aspartame is 180 to 200 times sweeter than sugar. The G. D. Searle Company sought FDA approval in 1973. The FDA approved it in 1974, but objections that aspartame might cause brain damage led to a stay, or legal postponement, of that approval. Another problem arose: an FDA investigation of records of animal studies conducted for Searle drug approvals and for aspartame raised questions. The FDA arranged for an independent audit, which took more than two years and concluded that the aspartame studies and results were authentic. The agency then organized an expert board of inquiry, whose members concluded that the evidence did not support the charge that aspartame might kill clusters of brain cells or cause other damage. However, persons with an inborn error of metabolism, phenylketonuria, must avoid protein foods such as meat that contain phenylalanine—one of the two components of aspartame. The board did, however, recommend that aspartame not be approved until further long-term animal testing could be conducted to rule out the possibility that aspartame might cause brain tumors. The FDA's Bureau of Foods viewed the study data then available and concluded that the board's concern was unfounded. Aspartame was approved for use as a tabletop sweetener in certain dry foods in 1981 and in soft drinks two years later.

In 1984 news reports, fueled by the announcement that the Arizona Department of Health Services was testing soft drinks containing aspartame to see if it deteriorated into toxic levels of methyl alcohol under storage conditions, created alarm. The Arizona health department acted after the director of the Food Sciences and Research Laboratory at Arizona State University submitted a study alleging that higher than normal temperatures could lead to a dangerous breakdown in the chemical composition.[45] The authors checked with representatives of the FDA, which said there are higher levels of methyl alcohol in regular fruit juices, so as far as the agency was concerned, the fears about decomposition were unfounded.

Questions also were raised about whether glutamic acid (see page 153) in combination with aspartame might contribute to brain damage, mental retardation, or hormone problems. The American Medical Association's Council on Scientific Affairs and the FDA have concluded that there is no evidence that aspartame, either alone or in combination with glutamate, can contribute to brain damage, mental retardation, or endocrine dysfunction.

The AMA council statement said: "Available evidence suggests that consumption of aspartame by normal humans is safe and is not as-

sociated with serious adverse health effects. Individuals who need to
control their phenylalanine intake should handle aspartame like any
other source of phenylalanine."[46]

Others are not so sure. Anecdotal reports of difficulties attributed to
the sweetener include painful menstruation, spotting between menstrual
periods, severe depression, dizziness, headaches, seizures, and birth defects. In 1986, the FDA refused to hold public hearings on the safety of
aspartame.[47] The FDA says it investigated two thousand cases of alleged
adverse effects from aspartame including eighty-five alleged epileptic
seizures. The agency concluded that of those complaints, seventeen may
possibly have been related to aspartame but that five of those seventeen
patients had a history of epilepsy.

Richard Wurtman, M.D., a professor of neuroendocrine regulation
at MIT, has conducted laboratory studies showing that aspartame,
given alone, nearly doubled central nervous system levels of phenylalanine in rats and quadrupled brain phenylalanine concentrations when
administered with glucose. The excess phenylalanine was converted to
tyrosine.[48]

Phenylalanine and tyrosine compete with other amino acids for transport across the blood-brain barrier, so the amino acid tryptophan was
significantly lower in the brains of rats that received glucose and aspartame than in those of control animals. Moreover, the calming neurotransmitter serotonin, manufactured from tryptophan, was similarly
decreased. Dr. Wurtman infers that people who ingest aspartame, especially in combination with carbohydrate snacks, may be in danger of
altering neurotransmission with unknown effects on emotion.

He says his studies show that the effect of the phenylalanine in the
brain doubles when aspartame and carbohydrates are combined. No one
knows what is a safe amount. There are several groups of people that
might be especially susceptible to such high doses. These include people
who are taking drugs that act on the brain (such as medications for high
blood pressure), people with a history of seizures, youngsters, and pregnant women. For adults who do not fall into the above categories, Dr.
Wurtman suggested that moderate amounts of aspartame a day should
not be hazardous.[49]

Since this artificial sweetener is not vital to well-being—except, perhaps, for some diabetics who have sweet cravings—you should ask yourself if it is really a necessity in your diet.

THE NERVOUS EXCITEMENT OF THE CHINESE RESTAURANT SYNDROME AND OTHER GLUTAMATES

Glutamate, a salt of the amino acid glutamic acid, is a remarkably potent, rapidly acting nerve toxin in laboratory cell cultures. It causes swelling of the nerve after only ninety seconds of contact.[50]

Why glutamate causes nerve injury is unknown. More than a decade ago it was believed that glutamate neurotoxicity is a direct consequence of overexciting nerves. More recently it has been thought that a calcium influx triggered by glutamate exposure might be involved in glutamate toxicity.[51] Under normal circumstances, the brain appears well equipped to handle large amounts of glutamate in harmless fashion, rapidly removing it and sequestering it away inside cells where it is nontoxic. In recent years, however, a number of disease states have been linked to glutamate neurotoxicity—among them, Huntington's disease, a hereditary brain-degenerating condition, and nerve loss associated with acute brain or spinal cord injury due to stroke or trauma, where injured nervous tissue may be unable to safely absorb glutamate and may, in addition, release glutamate from storage, leading to extension of the original injury.

It is now suspected that glutamate and related neurotransmitters may also be involved in the nerve tangles that form the brain cell degeneration found in Alzheimer's disease victims. Some researchers have demonstrated that in Alzheimer's disease there is a decrease in the brain receptors to which glutamate binds.

The cause of tangled nerve formations in Alzheimer's is still not understood, but the fact that such tangles are in the brain cells involved with processing glutamate raises interesting questions. Why are glutamate nerve cells susceptible to tangle formations? Is it a genetic abnormality, or do viruses invade this particular cell type? Both possibilities are intriguing. What if these neurons are producing abnormally high levels of glutamate, which could then act as a toxin? If this is true, the nerve degeneration associated with Alzheimer's disease might be halted with drugs that inhibit the effects of excess glutamate.[52]

MSG is the sodium of glutamic acid. It occurs naturally in seaweed, soybeans, and sugar beets. It is used commercially to intensify meat and spice flavorings in meats, condiments, pickles, soups, candies, and baked goods. It is believed responsible for the so-called Chinese restaurant syndrome, in which diners suffer from chest pain, headache, and numbness after eating a Chinese meal.

Some researchers believe that the Chinese restaurant syndrome is caused by a sudden elevation of glutamate in the blood which produces a blood vessel response. Another theory holds that some individuals have glutamate-sensitive receptors in the esophagus that can cause a heartburnlike reaction to MSG.[53]

MSG has been found to cause brain damage in young rodents and brain damage effects in rabbits, chicks, and monkeys. Baby-food processors removed MSG from its products. MSG is on the FDA list of additives that need further study for mutagenic, teratogenic, subacute, and reproductive effects. The final report in 1980 to the FDA of the Select Committee on Generally Recognized as Safe substances stated that while no evidence in the available information on MSG demonstrates a hazard to the public at current use levels, the uncertainties that exist require that additional studies be conducted. GRAS status continues while tests are being completed and evaluated.[54] But MSG is an unnecessary addition to food and, therefore, is not worth even the slightest risk.

WHAT IS BEING DONE TO PROTECT US FROM NEUROTOXINS?

Thomas J. Sobotka, Ph.D., of the Neurobehavioral Toxicology Team, Center for Food Safety and Applied Nutrition of the FDA, points out:

> The FDA must have a reasonable basis of scientific evidence to warrant any effective action. In making regulatory decisions about safety, agency personnel must consider any and all potentially adverse reactions. Traditionally, the agency has approached its evaluation of safety along the lines of conventional toxicology, considering such widely accepted indices of toxicity as mortality, pathology, carcinogenesis, growth disorders, clinical abnormalities, organ system impairment or failure, reproductive disorders, and teratogenic potential. Recently, however, there has been a growing opinion that such conventional measures of toxicity may not be sufficient to give a comprehensive profile of potential adverse effects of toxicants. The recognition that drugs, environmental chemicals and even dietary chemicals may influence the neuronal control of behavioral processes such as learning, attention, sensorimotor performance, sleep and

mood has generated considerable interest among the scientific and regulatory communities and concern among the general public. The realization that brain function may be influenced by such chemicals has spurred toxicologists to re-evaluate their conceptual definitions of toxicity to include the fact that changes in neuronal function may occur in conjunction with, prior to, or conceivably even in the absence of other signs of toxicity. What this means in terms of safety assessment is that the nature of the necessary database may have to be expanded not only to encompass measures of pathological toxicity but also to involve specific measures of brain dysfunction.[55]

Dr. Sobotka says that some neurotoxic testing occurs if there is a suspicion of central nervous system effects: "Typically, experimental animals are observed for any signs of neurotoxicity and the nervous system is studied at necropsy for pathology. There is no specific requirement for routine behaviorial testing but such testing may be requested if there is evidence of possible neurotoxicity. There is a difference between requiring a battery of behavioral tests for all chemicals as part of a toxicological screen and requiring such testing only for those chemicals for which there is some basis for asking specific questions about effects on the nervous system."[56]

He pointed out that the FDA is underfunded and understaffed, so that the burden of toxicological testing has to be with the industry. The FDA's Food Center has sixty-one toxicologists and an annual budget of $3,600,000.[57] By 1990, the food additive business alone is expected to be a $4.5-billion enterprise.[58]

Dr. Sobotka says that specialists in neurotoxicology are few and that there should be scientists who are specifically trained in neurotoxicology in both the FDA and in industry. But, he says, trained neurophysiologists are sharp enough to pick up on a problem if they are supplied with sufficient data. "A lot depends on the use level, the type of compound, and the amount of material that would eventually end up in foods," Dr. Sobotka continues. "Safety assessment must be comprehensive. In addition to toxicological effects such as cancer, which represents one of the most prominent health concerns, toxicologists must continue to be alert to numerous other forms of toxicity, including adverse effects to the functional integrity of organ systems such as the immune and nervous system."[59]

"One problem in doing functional assessment," he noted, "is that there are a number of factors that must be considered." He gave as an example the controlled studies of the Feingold Diet regimen: "There were a few children who reacted unusually to artificial colors but this result should not be taken out of context. The studies were with a highly select subgroup whose parents had already identified them as having attentional deficits. Avoiding artificial colors is not a solution to the hyperactive problem."[60]

As for aspartame and MSG, Dr. Sobotka says, "There is no reason to suspect that there is any problem with either, alone or in combination. It does appear some people are sensitive to monosodium glutamate and aspartame. It is fair to say that some individuals are going to react to some chemicals sometime in their lives. It is not an unusual occurrence. Therefore, the position to go for is use with moderation."[61]

According to Dr. Sobotka, while the FDA acknowledges that brain dysfunction is an important aspect of toxicology, there is no universal agreement as to how to incorporate this concern into the process of safety assessment. Some toxicologists question the very need for such tests. Other scientists feel that there is an inherent need to consider brain and behavior changes as well as conventional toxicology criteria. Dr. Sobotka says this attitude is based on the concern that, for some chemicals, nerve function changes may still occur at dose levels below which other signs of toxicity are evident.

He also points out that the FDA does not require specific neurobehavioral testing as part of its routine screen. However, the agency does have the authority to require such special neurobehavioral testing for any chemical substance if there is any evidence of nervous system involvement. The only time, then, that neurotoxicity is taken into account is when there is neuropathology or any obvious clinical sign of nerve damage, such as paralysis, tremor, or convulsion. Says Dr. Sobotka:

A credible and defensible regulatory decision must be supported by convincing evidence from valid studies that dietary exposure to a specific chemical or food ingredient either does or does not cause a defined behavioral dysfunction. In addition to clear cause-and-effect relationships, sufficient correlative information and supporting science must be available to enable the regulatory scientist to assess the relevance and significance of the observed nerve function effect[s], and to make predictions about the nature and size of the population at greatest risk for the toxicity.[62]

Absolute proof may take years to develop, however, especially in view of the fact that standardized testing methods for neurotoxins are almost nonexistent. L. Barry Goss, Ph.D., director of the environmental sciences department at Battelle Institute, points out that less than 10 percent of the seventy thousand chemicals in the marketplace have been tested to assess their risk to general human health and safety. Furthermore, other than the standard organophosphates (pesticides) gait test, there are no short-term tests that adequately assess the neurotoxicity of compounds. Says Dr. Goss, "Right now, chickens are given injections of an organophosphate and then a researcher watches the chicken as it walks to see if its gait is affected. If the chicken staggers around, then the researchers assume the compound has inhibited an enzyme in the brain, cholinesterase, involved in movement."[63]

Dr. Goss and his colleagues are working on neurotoxin tests involving simple organisms such as planeria and fish cells that can be done inexpensively in laboratory dishes and that will better determine a chemical's potential for damaging nerves. He said such tests could be coupled with behavioral tests in fish, for example, to screen for neurotoxins.[64]

The Chemical Industry Institute of Toxicology (CIIT), Research Triangle Park, North Carolina, founded in 1974 by the chemical industry, is also trying to develop new neurotoxicology tests. Dr. M. E. Pruitt, now a retired vice-president of the Dow Chemical Company and CIIT's first chairman, recently said: "by 1974, it became clear to many of us that much more toxicological data was needed on most chemicals."[65]

A CIIT position paper, released in April 1987,[66] said that many of the questions asked in 1974 are still unanswered. Among them:

- Which chemicals are dangerous, especially over long periods of time?
- How much exposure is too much?
- Are certain combinations of chemicals (or combinations of chemical exposure with certain elements of lifestyle, such as smoking or drinking) more dangerous than others?
- How can we identify in advance, rapidly and economically, chemicals that may cause problems?
- And, most important, how can the sum total of our observations of chemical toxicity be rationally compiled and analyzed so that the

informed decisions about the benefits of a compound versus its risks can be made?

The CIIT paper noted that among the "priority public issues" on which the current research program is now focusing are:

• Concern about reproductive and developmental or other adverse health effects from exposure to chemicals present in air, water, or food.

• The "emerging issue" of neurotoxicity.

Hugh A. Tilson, Ph.D, head of the neurobehavioral section of the National Institute of Environmental Health Sciences, Laboratory of Behavioral and Neurological Toxicology, in North Carolina, maintains that routine tests for nerve toxins should be included when screening food additives.

"We are not involved in the setting of regulations but provide data that might be used by an agency to determine whether there is toxicity present or not," he explains. "That data doesn't have to be used. The FDA currently has no guidelines for neurotoxicity tests and they should have."

Dr. Tilson says, "Such tests are simple and inexpensive and often could be done by technicians who now do other tests on animals. For example, studying the grip strength of animals and motor activity."[67]

Dr. Tilson points out that aspartame was extensively tested with routine toxicology tests and was shown to be a fairly innocuous substance. But what needs to be done is to take an animal population that is predisposed toward seizures and see if the chemical exacerbates an already existing propensity. If the chemical does the same in the human population predisposed to seizures, then people should be warned about ingesting it.

Dr. Tilson says that red flags about aspartame do exist. These are anecdotal reports about some people who say they experienced discomfort and some who reported having had actual seizures.

What are the potential risks to humans exposed to certain food chemicals before birth? What are the long-term consequences? Few tests are being done to answer these important questions.

The FDA's Dr. Sobotka agrees that there is a problem and that to evaluate the long-term effects of any compound is a problem for toxicology in general. Long-term effects on the brain and behavior are only now really being studied and evaluated. These kinds of studies are difficult to conduct because of the physiologic changes that occur with age.

Dr. Tilson believes that foods and drugs must be screened for neurotoxicity. As it stands now, the FDA requires no specific tests for neurotoxicity. They do do some neurotoxicity testing: a technician stands at the cage side and observes during the dosing period and notes any changes on a data sheet. This may not be sufficient. There should be a systematic series of observational tests that could be done on the animals during the course of exposure. Those tests should provide data that can be analyzed statistically in terms of whether or not there are any neurological signs. Many of these tests are relatively simple. If done properly, they can provide information about the degree of neurological dysfunction.

Such tests would involve performance of reflex tests, measures of muscle strength. The cost of the testing equipment would be about four- to five-thousand dollars per laboratory. When weighing costs, we must ask: what is the cost of treating a single individual whose brain has been damaged by a neurotoxin?

WHAT TO DO IN THE MEANTIME

- If you suspect you or a family member may be reacting adversely to food colorings, salicylates, or other food additives, try the Feingold Diet or just eliminate those foods with which you associate your symptoms. It can't hurt and it may help.

- Do not store acidic foods and beverages in lead-glazed ceramic ware or in cans. Consider storing such foods in glass containers if you have young children.

- Do not use aluminum cookware, if you have a choice, and do not use underarm deodorant sprays containing aluminum. Do not swallow digestion tablets containing the metal. Ration your intake of processed foods with aluminum (see list on pages 142–143).

- Avoid alcohol when you need your brain to work at its optimum— such as when driving, studying, or operating machinery. Even a little bit can dampen your intellect.

- Avoid alcohol and liquor in medications if you are pregnant or are taking any psychopharmaceuticals such as tranquilizers or antidepressants.

- Control your intake of caffeine, especially if you are pregnant or if you suffer from a great deal of anxiety.

- Skip the artificial sweeteners. There are troubling questions about aspartame and other artificial sweeteners. They are unnecessary— except perhaps for diabetics—and they do not really help with weight reduction. Pregnant women and children, especially, should avoid ingesting aspartame.

- Do not add the flavor enhancer MSG to your foods. It is an unnecessary and questionable ingredient, especially when the meal also contains aspartame (see page 153).

- Write to your legislators and insist that additives be tested for neurotoxicity prior to being added to our food. Foods that may be contaminated with neurotoxic pollutants should be identified and removed from the market.

⊰ 9 ⊱

Building a Child's Brain Power
with Food

T hirty-two-year-old Kathy, in her twenty-ninth week of pregnancy, was admitted to the hospital in Baltimore for observation of a skin rash and hives that developed after she had eaten steamed crabs and cherries. Her blood pressure was low and she was having contractions every two to three minutes. Her baby's heartbeat was slow and irregular.

Once the physicians determined that the baby's distress was secondary to Kathy's food allergy, the doctors gave Kathy oxygen, intravenous fluids, and a standard dose of antihistamines to fight the allergic attack. Kathy's labor contractions stopped and her baby's heartbeat returned to normal within two hours. Eleven and a half uneventful weeks later, she delivered a healthy boy whose intelligence and reflexes were normal.[1]

This case illustrates that what a pregnant woman eats can directly affect her unborn child.

Animal experiments have demonstrated that a fetus can even taste and smell the food that is passed to it from its mother. Taste buds are among the earliest sense organs to appear in the fetus, according to Charlotte M. Mistretta of the University of Michigan in Ann Arbor. She and her colleagues performed experiments on sheep fetuses delivered by cesarean section and still connected to their mothers by the umbilical cord. The researchers found that by the third trimester of pregnancy, fetal taste buds were responsive to chemicals in the amniotic fluid and that the taste responses changed substantially during subsequent fetal development. Taste buds of third-trimester sheep fetuses responded to a variety of flavors, and those responses produced detectible electrical signals in their brains, Mistretta reported. Early in the third trimester, the fetal taste

161

buds reacted to ammonium chloride but not to table salt. The fetuses
gradually increased their responses to sodium as they developed.[2]

The sense of smell also appears to function before birth. Yale researchers injected an odorous substance into amniotic fluid around rat fetuses
and found that the odor affected the sucking behavior of the rats after
birth.[3]

A human unborn baby, then, presumably can taste and smell the food
it is offered. But what can it do if it doesn't like the menu offered in the
uterus? A fetus is a parasite. It can't get up and go out to the supermarket
and select its own diet. And yet, there is no time in human life when the
brain is more vulnerable to the effects of food than in the womb.

Interference with the orderly sequence of brain development can not
only cause physical changes in the brain but also affect behavior and
intellect. A great deal of experimentation with animals and observation
of children who are undernourished indicate that the consequences of
poor nutrition before and soon after birth in intellectual ability and
behavior are dependent on the nature, severity, time during development, and duration of the nutritional deprivation.[4]

Nutritional insults can be devastating if they occur during the brain
growth spurt, which in human babies extends from the second trimester
of pregnancy to the age of two years. This is a critical period of development in which the organ's growth is most rapid. The increase in cells and
the formation of the connections between brain cells makes the baby's
brain most vulnerable to diet at this time. Nerve cells form according to
a complex programmed chronology of events; insults inflicted at a particular time may interfere with specific nerve cell types.

Undernourished babies during this period have brains that are lighter
in weight and a decrease in the number and size of cells, total protein
and fat content, and thickness of the cerebral cortex—the "thinking
brain." If the nutritional deprivation occurs early in life and the baby has
a fewer number of brain cells, the deficit is permanent. A later insult
reduces cell size and is reversible.

The amount of *myelin* deposited is reduced in undernourished babies.
The myelin sheath functions as an insulator for the electrical impulses
conducted along nerves. If it is deficient, "static" occurs when nerve
messages are sent and such brain functions as movement, speech, and
thinking are affected.[5]

For the brain to function normally, not only must there be an appropriate number of brain cells with well-placed connections, but also brain nerve cells must be able to manufacture and release neurotransmitters. The latter relay impulses between nerve cells which have synapses between them. Nutrition, as we have pointed out again and again in this book, affects neurotransmitter production.

Protein malnutrition can impair behavior by reducing the ability to think clearly and by affecting motivation and social characteristics. Some researchers believe that malnutrition in children does not need to produce obvious lesions in the brain to affect intellect, behavior, and learning. The action may be indirect. Undernutrition may interfere with the ability to concentrate during critical periods of development and lead to motivational and personality changes, any one of which may impair learning *performance* rather than learning *capacity*.

This was shown when animal fetuses were given a known neurotoxin, *methylazoxymethanol* (MAM). The type of nerve damage caused by MAM in the brains of the unborn animals looked just like that seen in the brains of mentally ill adults during autopsies. Early investigations show that animals exposed to MAM before birth were similar to controls in most measures of learning, although some substantial deficits were seen in maze learning. MAM-treated animals were found to be hyperactive. More recently, it has been shown that prenatal treatment with MAM causes marked changes in the production of neurotransmitters in the brain. These findings provide further support for the idea that prenatal administration of MAM may constitute a method of altering brain structure comparable to the kinds of damage thought to be responsible for some human psychiatric disorders.[6]

Nature has protected the human fetus by surrounding it in the womb with a nourishing fluid that keeps it safe. Part of that protection is the ability of the unborn baby to be selfish and take nutrients from the mother, even if it makes the mother deficient. According to Herman Baker, Ph.D.,

> If you look at the blood of a mother during pregnancy and then you take a sample of the blood from the umbilical cord, you will find that the baby usually has about three to five times more circulating vitamins than the mother, except for vitamin A and vitamin E. There the ratio is usually reversed. If the mother starts her pregnancy off as vitamin deficient, the baby will be born vitamin deficient. Whatever effect this has on growth and intellectual development, we still don't know the entire picture.[7]

Scientists do know that one element missing from many pregnant women's diets is iodine (see page 54), and this deficiency is believed to be the factor most responsible worldwide for brain damage in children. Iodine is needed for the function of the thyroid gland. In early pregnancy, the fetus is apparently dependent on its mother's thyroid hormone. After the fetal thyroid develops, the baby makes its own. A lack of thyroid hormone during brain development impairs cell division, growth, and the formation of synapses between nerve cells, and suppresses the myelination (covering) of nerves. A woman's iodine-deficient diet during pregnancy can result in severe retardation of her child or a milder syndrome of physical incoordination, with or without some deficit in intelligence. The most severe illness is known as cretinism, in which there is mental retardation, physical incoordination, deafness, and, in some cases, dwarfism.[8]

The similarity of these abnormalities to those that occur in zinc deficiency supports the concept that deficiency of any nutrient critical for brain development can disrupt the well-ordered maturation of the brain. When a mother does not have enough zinc in her diet, it has been shown in animal experiments in the United States and Europe, there is an adverse effect on the behavior of the offspring after birth.[9] It is believed that this effect is due to the zinc deficiency causing changes in the levels of serotonin and other brain neurotransmitters.[10]

Zinc is essential for the activity of many enzymes. Hence, various investigators support the association of zinc deficiency as a factor in birth defects of the brain. Development of the "smell" center of the brain is abnormal in many zinc-deficient animal fetuses, and the fetuses frequently have hydrocephalus (water on the brain). A statistical difference has also been found between zinc levels in the blood of babies born with small brains compared to those of normal babies.[11] Furthermore, in children, insufficient levels of zinc have been associated with lower learning ability, apathy, lethargy, and mental retardation.

A manganese-deficient diet in pregnant mice and guinea pigs has shown that this micronutrient may be essential for the brains of unborn human babies. When animal mothers had a diet deficient in manganese, their babies staggered after they were born. This condition was due to impaired formation of the inner-ear mechanisms involved in balance. The problem can be prevented by feeding pregnant rats and guinea pigs one milligram of manganese per gram of diet. In addition to impairing inner-ear development, manganese deficiency has also been reported to lower the neurotransmitter content of the brain. Although manganese deficiency-induced behavioral abnormalities in humans have not been described, behavioral effects of manganese overdoses are well known. Manganese poisoning in miners has resulted in Parkinson's disease, a common disorder of the part of the brain that controls movement, and demented behavior due to accumulation of the element in the brain.[12]

THE DRINK THAT GOES RIGHT TO
AN UNBORN BABY'S HEAD

Alcoholic beverages are the most common cause in the western world of damage to the brains of unborn children from something their mothers consume. It is estimated that as many as two percent of all live births may show effects of alcohol exposure on the fetus. Prenatal exposure to alcohol affects the development of various systems, including those of the muscles, skeleton, and nerves. Many infants with fetal alcohol syndrome have symptoms that point to abnormal development of the brain, particularly of the areas that control movement and speech. Such abnormalities include muscle weakness, incoordination, and difficulties with language and thinking. Anatomical studies of the brains of mature humans who had been exposed to alcohol before birth show that their brains are smaller and that the organization of their brains' nerve cells is abnormal.[13]

As little as one alcoholic drink a day in early pregnancy can adversely affect an unborn child's growth. In a recent study, researchers in London enrolled 144 pregnant women in a program to examine factors predictive of birth weight.[14] The study found that regular drinkers gave birth to infants who weighed at least 700 grams less than the infants of infrequent drinkers. The analysis suggested that drinking an average of one drink daily before the first prenatal visit decreased the birth weight of boy infants by an average of 230 grams and the weight of girl infants by an average of 25 grams. The well-documented effects of mothers' excessive drinking on their offspring include growth deficiencies, specific facial deformities, and brain dysfunction that may be related to abnormal brain development. And although alcohol can be harmful to the fetus at any time during pregnancy, researchers believe that the most toxic effect on the development of the human nervous system is relatively late in pregnancy, particularly during the final three months.[15]

Incidently, alcohol is present in more than seven hundred prescribed liquid medications, many of them teething preparations, decongestants, and cough medicines. So read labels carefully if you are pregnant or if you want to give even an over-the-counter medication to your child. Ethanol affects children's bodies more rapidly than it does adults, and children are more susceptible to its effects, which include central nervous system impairment, decreased reaction time, muscle incoordination, and behavioral changes.[16]

TAKE THE MILK AND SKIP
THE COFFEE, TEA, AND COLAS

Caffeine is another common ingredient in drinks and medicine that, when ingested by a pregnant woman, can go right to her unborn child's head. In order to study the effects of caffeine ingested by the pregnant mother on the development of her offspring, scientists at the Hebrew University in Rehovot, Israel, administered caffeine to pregnant rats by mixing it with drinking water during the last seven days of pregnancy.[17] This is a period of rapid development, roughly equivalent to the rapid development during mid-pregnancy in humans. Three groups of pregnant rats were treated with varying doses of caffeine. One group was given a dose roughly equivalent to four cups of coffee per day for seven days. The second group was given eight cups per day and the third about twelve cups per day. The pups born to these three groups of rats were followed from birth well into adulthood and were compared on various measures of physical and behavioral development to the pups born to rat mothers that did not receive caffeine.

The results showed that the lowest dose of caffeine (equal to about four cups of coffee daily) caused hyperactivity in the offspring but no serious learning problems. However, the animals whose mothers were treated with the two higher doses (equal to about eight and twelve cups of coffee daily) showed learning deficits on complex learning tasks where sustained attention was necessary for success in the task. The learning disability was more marked in the animals exposed to the highest doses. In addition to learning deficits, the animals exposed to the two higher doses of caffeine before birth were significantly more obese in adulthood than those in the low-dose group or the non-caffeine-treated control group. Both the obesity and the learning disability became more severe with increasing age.

WHAT TO EAT AND WHAT NOT TO EAT IF YOU ARE PREGNANT

It would be best for your baby's brain if you avoided ingestion of all alcoholic and caffeinated beverages. Such libations are unnecessary, and while a minimum amount may do no harm, why take any risk at all? Remember that colas, chocolate, and medicines may contain caffeine. Medicines may also have alcohol.

A pregnant woman should, of course, have medical supervision during gestation. Those who have a family history of diabetes or high blood pressure must follow a carefully monitored diet. Diabetes and high blood pressure often make their first appearance during the physical stress of pregnancy. However, for healthy women without medical problems, there are still special needs, particularly for calcium, iodine, and certain vitamins. Chapter 3 provides information about specific nutrients. The table shown on the next page outlines a prudent general diet for a healthy, pregnant woman and her unborn child.

GOOD NUTRITION FOR A NEWBORN

In recent years, scientists have discovered that nerve regulation systems are organized differently in the young than in the adult. Additionally, there may be two or three transitional stages *after* birth. The interaction of a mother and her baby have been found to regulate certain aspects of the infant's nervous system development. For example, it has been found in rats that the rate and quality of milk provided by the mother regulates autonomic nervous system development in the infant. There is also evidence that touch and smell stimulation may serve to regulate the behavior responses of the infant by affecting the accumulation of brain neurotransmitters.[18] These are additional reasons that a human child should be breast-fed if at all possible. If not, then a mother should hold and cuddle her baby during bottle-feeding.

Breast-feeding provides the ideal nourishment for human babies. The

FOOD	FIRST FOUR MONTHS	SECOND FIVE MONTHS
High-calcium foods such as yogurt, milk, cheese, and ice cream	2–4 servings per day	4 servings per day
Protein foods such as chicken, fish, meat, beans, and peanut butter	2 servings per day	3 servings per day
Vegetables (dark-green or deep-yellow) such as spinach, broccoli, squash, and carrots	1–2 servings per day	1–2 servings per day
Citrus fruits or juices such as orange juice (fresh squeezed)	1–2 servings per day	2 servings per day
Breads, cereals, and pastas (whole-grain or enriched)	3 servings per day	4–5 servings per day

protein content of breast milk is particularly suited to a baby's metabolism, and the fat content is more easily absorbed and digested than that in cow's milk. Because it contains antibodies from the mother, breast milk can also provide immunity against certain infections and allergies.

There is more vitamin A and vitamin E and twice as much iron in human milk, which may protect against anemia in the baby and thus protect the red blood cells that carry oxygen to the baby's brain. Zinc and taurine, an amino acid that not only aids in digestion but also is thought to be important in brain and nervous system development, are also more available in breast milk.[19]

Milk production requires a lot of energy. Women who eat a healthy diet while they are pregnant and stay within the number of calories recommended by their doctors usually gain about eight to ten pounds of fat—about a third more than they had before they became pregnant. This extra store of fat is nature's assurance there will be sufficient calories available to produce enough milk after the baby is born. A healthy breast-feeding diet is basically the same nutritionally sound and varied diet recommended during pregnancy. The main differences are the needs for extra calories, fluids, and certain vitamins.[20]

Exactly how many calories should a breast-feeding mother eat? The National Academy of Sciences recommends that a woman who is five-feet, four-inches tall and weighs about 120 pounds should eat 2,600 calories a day while nursing. This is in comparison to a recommended 2,400 calories a day while pregnant and 2,100 calories a day when neither pregnant nor nursing.[21]

Yet a mother can have a poor diet—either nutritionally inadequate or too low in calories or both—and still produce milk for her baby. This is especially true during the first few months of breast-feeding, when the extra fat from pregnancy is available. As those fat reserves are depleted, the amount of milk produced may decrease.

But remember: what a mother ingests may be passed through the breast milk to the baby, affecting the baby's brain and body. Alcohol, for example, passes easily into breast milk. Large amounts of beer or wine can make your baby drunk, affect his coordination and emotions, and lead to dehydration. Caffeine reaches the breast milk in smaller amounts, but if you ingest enough caffeine, your baby may become irritable and have trouble sleeping.

Recreational drugs, of course, should not be taken at all. Prescription drugs and over-the-counter medications, even such common ones as antihistamines and painkillers, should not be taken unless prescribed by a doctor. If a medicine works, it has a systemic effect—that is, it affects your entire body. If it has a systemic effect, it may affect the unborn child.

Each mother's breast milk is custom designed for her baby with antibodies and other ingredients, including the amino acid taurine, which is one hundred times greater in human than in cow's milk. The milk changes from day to day. The mother of a premature infant, for example, will have a higher fat content in her milk than a mother who has given birth to a full-term baby. Premature infants needs the higher fat content.[22]

There are more than one hundred ingredients in human milk that are not in cow's milk. Your baby may grow faster and heavier on cow's milk because of the added calcium it contains, but bigger is not necessarily better.

In the western world, where many mothers work outside the home, it may not be feasible to breast-feed. Most children will thrive on a formula. Whenever possible, however, breast-feeding is preferable.

The following page outlines a nutritious diet for breast-feeding mothers.

For a variety of reasons, baby or weaning foods should not be given until the infant is four to six months old. One reason is that the younger baby's system is not prepared to handle such food. The Committee on Nutrition of the American Academy of Pediatrics points out that the infant's digestive system is not prepared to cope with the proteins contained in foods other than breast milk or formula. Also, before the age of four to six months, the kidneys are not mature enough to deal with the concentrated amounts of protein, minerals, and electrolytes present in solid food. Moreover, an infant has difficulty simply recognizing a spoon and coordinating the movements of chewing and swallowing. A young baby isn't able to signal his mother whether he is hungry or full. All of these abilities require further development of the nervous system. Thus, giving solid foods to an infant amounts to force-feeding.[23]

FOOD FOR THE GROWING CHILD'S BRAIN

Human studies have shown that even a mildly undernourished child can affect a mother-child relationship. The malnourished child who is apathetic and unresponsive to the mother's attentions elicits less response or stimulation from the mother. This, in turn, can affect the child's behavior and learning ability.

It is difficult to separate direct effects of malnutrition on the brain and the effect of malnutrition on the ability to receive information. Malnourished children show decreased motivation, concentration, and attentiveness, which may impair successful learning. Undernutrition, therefore, is a significant nongenetic factor influencing the development of the brain in unborn and young children.

Severe malnutrition, not only in the first few months of life but any time within the first two years, has long-lasting consequences on cognitive development. Jamaican boys who were severely malnourished during the first two years of life had lower intelligence scores and decreased intellectual ability compared with their brothers, sisters, and classmates.[24]

A short exposure to malnutrition in a previously well-nourished popu-

BREAST-FEEDING DIET

FOOD	AMOUNT
Fluids	*6 to 8 glasses per day*
Milk	
Fruit juices	
Water	
Proteins	*Two servings per day*
Lean meat, poultry, fish, or cheese	3 oz.
Nuts, seeds, or cottage cheese	4 oz.
Peanut butter, pasta, dried beans, or peas	8 oz.
Eggs	2
Calcium Sources	*Enough to total 850 mg. per day*
Milk, yogurt	1 cup = 215 mg.
Cheese	1½ oz. = 50–400 mg., depending on type
Salmon or sardines	3 oz. salmon = 167 mg.; 3 oz. sardines = 372 mg.
Ice cream	1 cup = about 190 mg.
Dried beans	3 cups cooked = 25–120 mg. (depending on type)
Kale	1 cup cooked = 210 mg.
Broccoli	1 cup cooked = 140 mg.
Tofu	2½ × 2¼ × 1-inch piece = 150 mg.
Breads and Cereals (Carbohydrates)	*Four servings per day*
Whole-grain bread	1 slice = 24 mg.
Cooked oat or rice cereal	½ cup = 22 mg.
Wheat germ	1 tablespoon = 3 mg.
Pasta	1 cup cooked = 11 mg.
Crackers	4 saltines = 6 mg.
Rice	1 cup cooked = 34 mg.

lation may not have lasting effects. This was shown in males born during the Dutch famine of 1944–45, who at eighteen years of age had scores on intelligence tests similar to controls from nonfamine areas.[25] As the intelligence tests were not performed until the subjects were eighteen years old, however, it is not known whether an initial deficit in intelligence resulted from the nutritional insult.

Kwashiorkor, infantile pellagra, is a malignant malnutrition due particularly to a lack of protein in the diet. *Marasmus* is a wasting disease found especially in young children and due to prolonged dietary deficiency of protein and calories. Studies of mental performance of kwashiorkor patients during the period of rehabilitation have shown that as children recover from malnutrition, developmental quotients increase in most cases. The magnitude of the increment was in direct relation to the age at which the children suffered the disease. Therefore, with successful treatment, the difference between chronological and mental age progressively diminished in all children except in those who were stricken by severe malnutrition below the age of six months.[26]

Research conducted on children recovering from marasmus or kwashiorkor show that they behave in similar ways and may be retarded in mental and physical development even after they become well-fed.

Joaquin Cravioto, M.D., professor of pediatrics and scientific director of the National Institute for Children's Health Sciences and Technology, Mexico City, a world-famous expert on the effects of malnutrition on children's brains, believes the deficits caused by malnutrition need not be permanent. In a 1981 lecture, Dr. Cravioto maintained that a good mother-child interaction after a child has been nutritionally rehabilitated can bring the majority of such children back to normal age levels of performance.[27]

Dr. Cravioto and his colleagues measured the mental performance of children who had suffered from malnutrition and were then well nourished.[28] The results showed that children who recovered from malnutrition had significantly lower intellectual quotients than their brothers, sisters, and other healthy children of the same social class. The children who had received stimulation during the period of hospitalization, however, had higher levels of performance than the group without stimulation, which proved the importance of nonnutritional variables such as cuddling and playing. Therefore, providing systematic stimulation to infants at high risk of developing severe malnutrition can diminish the negative effects on mental development and performance caused by this syndrome.

Dr. Cravioto says that the disappearance of the developmental lag in the survivors points to the strong association among nutrition, stimulation available at home, and brain function. Nutrition plays a major role in some brain functions and stimulation may influence another set of brain functions.

"We are beginning to tease out the differences related to nutritional insult either alone or in combination with other nonnutritional components of the environment of the malnourished children. We are just moving into the problem of scientifically defining the development sequence at which quantitative estimated levels of nutritional deficiency may interfere with emerging functions to give either delayed or disordered development,"[29] says Dr. Cravioto.

Derek Bryce-Smith, Ph.D., chairman of the Department of Organic Chemistry, University of Reading, England, has observed that in general, the development of nerve connections appears to involve two distinct processes that involve "hard" and "soft" wiring. The blueprint for the former appears to be programmed in some utterly mysterious ways into the structure of the developing brain, or even the fertilized egg, and the complex pattern of connections appear to be independent of input from the various senses. In contrast, the soft wiring is subject to alterations in, if not controlled by, the senses after birth. For example, rats that were frequently handled and placed in a stimulating environment showed increased brain weight and nerve connections and changes in brain chemistry, compared with rats kept on the same diet in a dull and unstimulating environment. Thus, brain development can be promoted both by social stimulus and by chemical stimulus, as with protein and zinc.[30]

FOOD FOR THE GROWING BRAIN

A child has special dietary requirements because of rapid growth. A reduced version of an adult diet is not sufficient. Youngsters have an increased need for calories and for all nutrients, one of the most important of which is iron. Iron-deficiency anemia is the most common nutritional deficiency problem in the United States.[31]

Folic acid, vitamin B_{12}, and copper are also important in making red blood cells. Protein is necessary for bone and cell growth, including nerve cells in the brain, and calcium is vital for building strong bones and teeth during childhood and adolescence. Some experts believe the RDA's for calcium should be increased to 1,000 to 1,200 milligrams per day for children.

RECOMMENDED DAILY DIETARY ALLOWANCES FOR CHILDREN

AGE (IN YEARS)	PROTEIN grams	CALCIUM milligrams	IRON milligrams	CALORIES
1–3	23[a]	800	15	900–1,800
4–6	30	800	10	1,300–2,300
7–10	34	800	10	1,650–3,300
11–14 (boys)	45	800	18	2,000–3,700
11–14 (girls)	46	1,200	18	1,500–3,000
15–18 (boys)	56	1,200	18	2,100–3,900
15–18 (girls)	46	1,200	18	1,200–3,000

[a] 1 oz. = approximately 28 grams.
SOURCE: Food and Nutrition Board, National Academy of Sciences—National Research Council, Recommended Daily Dietary Allowances Revised 1980

FAT TRAPS FOR CHILDREN

We described anorexia and bulimia in chapter 00. Data published in the May 1987 *American Journal of Diseases of Children* by a Boston team headed by Dr. Steven L. Gortmaker of the Harvard University School of Public Health show that since the mid-1960s, among children six to eleven years of age, obesity has become 54 percent more common and "super-obesity" has become 98 percent more common.[32] Adolescents are also fatter today, the team found, with a 39-percent increase in obesity and a 64-percent increase in super-obesity among those twelve to seventeen years of age. The Harvard researchers define an obese child as one having a body-fat thickness that is at or above the eight-fifth percentile for all children his or her age. Super-obesity, they said, is fatness at or above the ninety-fifth percentile. So a child is considered obese if 84 percent of his age-mates have smaller layers of fat on their frames. While added pounds may have an indirect effect on brain physiology, obesity has psychological consequences that affect brain function.

Treating obese children is difficult not only because it requires controlling their eating habits but because they have special dietary needs that must be met for proper growth.

The recommendations for children's diets are controversial, even among such illustrious groups as the American Heart Association, the American Cancer Society, and the American Academy of Pediatrics. The National Institutes of Health, the American Heart Association, and the American Cancer Society recommend lowering the amount of fat in children's diet, but the American Academy of Pediatrics finds "no compelling new evidence" that current diets should be modified. The pediatricians set the acceptable upper limits of fat intake in children at 40 percent of total calories.[33] The pediatricians questioned whether diets such as those recommended by the National Institutes of Health would adequately support growth, especially during the adolescent growth spurt:

> The safety of diets designed to decrease intake of refined sugars, decrease consumption of fat and cholesterol, and limit sodium intake has not been established in growing children and pregnant women. An increase in cereal grains at the expense of animal protein with a decrease in the density of essential nutrients without further dietary advice might result in a decrease of some protective micronutrients such as vitamins and minerals that might pose health risks to children.[34]

The August 1987 issue of the journal *Pediatrics* carried a caution to parents who are "overly concerned" about their infants' diets. A study of seven infants referred to North Shore University Hospital in Manhasset, New York, from 1981 to 1985, reported that these children of college-educated parents failed to thrive. The babies had decreased growth and poor weight gain. Michael Pugliese, M.D., and Fima Lifshitz, M.D., said in the study that the parents perceived these children as being similar to themselves—that is, obese, prone to atherosclerosis, and chronically dieting to reduce weight. These restrictive diets, however, typically including lean meats, low-fat dairy foods, and complex carbohydrates—foods already present in the parents' diets—caused the infants to experience inadequate weight gain and have a decreased linear growth rate. The infants were consuming only 60 to 94 percent of the recommended calorie intake for age and sex.[35] Whether this study stands the test of time or whether the slower growth and weight gain may not be as undesirable as the pediatricians believe, is yet to be determined.

Many experts disagree with the American Academy of Pediatrics dietary recommendations and point out that hardening of the arteries, which affects not only the heart but also the brain, begins in childhood. In a study reported in the January 1986 issue of the *New England Journal of Medicine,* researchers at Louisiana State University Medical Center reported that the earliest stages of heart disease were found in teen-agers who had high total cholesterol levels in their blood and high levels of the dangerous LDL cholesterol (see pages 96–97). The study was done on thirty-five youngsters, with an average age of 18 years, who died unexpectedly and who had been tested previously for cholesterol. All but six of them had "fatty streaks," thought to be precursors of fibrous cholesterol lesions, in their aortas, the artery that carries blood from the heart to the brain and the rest of the body.[36]

The concept that fat children outgrow their obesity is not based on the weight of evidence. Forty percent of children who are obese at age seven years become obese adults. And 70 percent of obese adolescents become obese adults.[37]

One provocative hypothesis is that the increased incidence of obesity in this country over the past twenty years was caused, at least in part, by television. William Dietz of the New England Medical Center Hospitals in Boston, reports that his studies have led him to this conclusion: "There was a strong, significant relationship between television viewing and obesity that persisted even when we introduced control after control."[38]

"Children eat more while they are watching TV and they eat more of the foods advertised on TV," Dietz says. "The message that TV conveys is that you will be thin no matter what you eat. Nearly everyone on television is thin. In addition, children who are watching television are inactive."

Dietz is now starting studies of the metabolic rates of children while they watch television. The first child he looked at, a 12 year old boy, had a basal metabolic rate that dropped by 200 calories an hour while he watched cartoons, as though he was in a trance or stupor.[39]

A. W. Logue, Ph.D., associate professor in the psychology department at the State University of New York at Stony Brook, says in her text *The Psychology of Eating and Drinking* that television is one of the clearest examples of the indirect influence of one organism on the food preferences of another.

> Children living in the United States view an average of some 22,000 commercials a year, and more than 50% of these advertised foods that are low in nutrition. . . . Several experiments have shown that when children are exposed to commercials for low-nutrition foods, their reported preference for those foods as well as their tendency to buy or eat those foods increases. On the other hand, when children are exposed to commercials that present nutritional information, their preference for nutritive foods is not affected. To some extent these differential results may be due to the greater amount of effort and money that is put into producing low-nutrition food commercials, compared with commercials carrying nutritional information. Nevertheless, the implications of this research are alarming. Most of the commercials that are seen by children appear to be teaching the children to prefer low-nutrition foods.[40]

WHAT ABOUT SUGAR?

One of the major objections regarding television and diet as far as children are concerned is that the commercials urge youngsters to eat highly sugared foods, particularly breakfast cereals and candy. Here are the results of Dr. Bette Li's testing of the sugar content of breakfast cereals, including granola cereals touted as "natural and healthy." Dr. Li and her colleagues Priscilla Schuhmann and Joanne Holden are with the Nutrient Composition Laboratory of the U.S. Department of Agriculture, Beltsville, Maryland.

Human and animal experiments have linked sugar and unruly behavior in children. A study found significant correlations between carbohydrate-protein ratios and directly observed aggressive and restless behavior in a sample of twenty-eight hyperactive children.[41] An estimation of sugar intake based on large categories of food also was associated with the same behaviors in the hyperactive group. Among the normal control children, the dietary carbohydrate-protein ratio correlated only with restless behavior. However, the study did not prove that sugar caused the hyperactivity or aggressiveness. It could be that active or aggressive children simply crave more sugar.

PRODUCT	FRUCTOSE	GLUCOSE	LACTOSE	MALTOSE	SUCROSE	TOTAL SUGAR
All Bran	1.09–1.64	0.90– 0.98	ND[a]	1.32–1.54	15.6 –16.0	19.3 –19.4
Apple Jacks	0.21–0.32	0.27– 0.42	ND	ND	52.4 –55.6	52.4 –55.6
Cocoa Krispies	0.32–0.39	0.77– 0.85	0.72–0.82	ND	39.0 –43.8	40.8 –45.8
Concentrate	0.20–0.30	0.03– 0.11	ND	ND	8.45–10.2	8.65–10.6
Corn Flakes	1.02–1.20	1.15– 1.34		<.1 –0.50	2.17– 2.65	4.80– 5.21
	1.08–1.18	1.16– 1.58		0.35–0.40	2.23– 3.33	5.39– 6.05
Corny Snaps	0.19–0.30	0.20– 0.35	ND	ND	35.1 –45.4	35.7 –45.8
Cracklin' Bran	0.64–0.70	1.23– 1.52	ND	0.82–0.96	25.3 –28.7	28.4 –31.8
Froot Loops	ND	ND	ND	ND	47.7 –49.1	47.7 –49.1
Frosted Mini Wheats	ND	ND	ND	ND	25.0 –26.1	25.0 –26.1
Frosted Rice	0.59–0.83	0.76– 1.02	ND	ND	32.4 –37.4	33.8 –39.2
Product 19	0.84–0.94	0.82– 0.91	ND	ND	7.84– 8.36	9.53–10.0
Raisin Bran	9.36–9.51	7.87– 8.23	ND	ND	11.4 –11.6	28.7 –29.4
Rice Krispies	0.38–0.53	0.30– 0.44	ND	ND	6.9 – 7.3	6.9 – 7.3
Special K	0.24–0.30	0.22– 0.24			4.85– 4.99	4.85– 4.99
	0.23–0.25	0.19– 0.24			4.58– 5.20	5.03– 5.68
Sugar Corn Pops	1.02–1.21	5.60– 6.32	ND	ND	37.6 –40.2	44.4 –47.6
Sugar Frosted Flakes	0.72–0.93	0.89– 1.03	ND	ND	35.8 –42.0	37.5 –43.6
Sugar Smacks	1.23–1.34	11.3 –11.8	ND	ND	41.4 –44.0	53.9 –57.1

NOTE: Reprinted, with permission, from Betty Li and P. J. Schuhmann, *Journal of Food Science,* Vol. 45 (1980). The detection limit was 0.01 percent for fructose and glucose and 0.1 percent for lactose, maltose, and sucrose.

[a]ND = Not detectable.

PRODUCT	MANUFACTURER	FRUCTOSE	GLUCOSE	LACTOSE	SUCROSE	TOTAL SUGAR
Country Morning	Kellogg	3.32–4.97	4.24–5.46	3.01–3.69	17.3–19.3	29.7–31.5
C.W. Post, Plain	General Foods	0.74	1.59–1.64	2.62–3.26	19.1–19.9	24.1–25.8
C.W. Post, Raisin	General Foods	2.36–3.06	3.12–3.86	1.89–2.60	19.0–19.2	27.2–28.6
Familia	Bio-Familia A.G.	3.35–4.47	2.20–3.31	ND[a]	15.4–18.4	22.6–24.5
Heartland, Coconut	Pet	1.60–1.68	1.87–1.90	ND	18.1–19.3	21.6–22.9
Heartland, Raisin	Pet	3.38–4.10	3.58–4.26	ND	17.8–18.9	25.1–26.8
Nature Valley Granola Cinnamon and Raisin	General Mills	2.70–5.31	2.42–4.84	ND	17.2–18.1	23.2–27.3
Nature Valley Granola Fruit and Nut	General Mills	3.07–4.73	3.86–6.71	ND	19.4–21.5	28.4–30.5
Quaker 100% Natural, Apple and Cinnamon	Quaker Oats	2.48–4.96	1.05–1.93	1.92–2.26	17.9–18.2	23.4–26.7
Quaker 100% Natural, Brown sugar and Honey	Quaker Oats	0.49–0.78	0.29–0.61	2.39–2.79	17.5–18.4	21.4–21.9
Quaker 100% Natural, Raisins and dates	Quaker Oats	3.53–5.88	5.10–8.12	2.50–2.69	14.7–16.2	26.1–31.6
Vita Crunch, Almond	Organic Milling	0.63–3.14	0.58–2.85	ND	23.8–25.9	26.0–29.8
Vita Crunch, Raisin	Organic Milling	0.57–2.83	0.63–2.54	ND	21.8–24.3	25.2–29.6
Vita Crunch, Regular	Organic Milling	0.16–0.46	0.16–0.45	ND	22.4–24.3	23.1–24.6

NOTE: Reprinted, with permission, from Betty Li and P. J. Schuhmann, *Journal of Food Science,* Vol. 45 (1980).
[a]ND = Not detectable. The detection limit was 0.4 percent for lactose.

PRODUCT	FRUCTOSE	GLUCOSE	LACTOSE	MALTOSE	SUCROSE	TOTAL SUGAR
Alphabits	< 0.5	< 0.5	ND[a]	ND	35.4 –39.9	35.4 –39.9
Bran Flakes, 40 percent	0.85–1.32	0.76–1.17	ND	0.75–1.22	9.22–10.7	11.6 –14.4
C. W. Post, Plain	0.61–0.76	1.64–1.83	1.69–1.86	2.61–4.72	19.7 –20.4	27.1 –28.5
C. W. Post, Raisin	3.84–5.48	4.28–5.90	1.22–1.26	ND	18.1 –18.5	27.4 –31.1
Cocoa Pebbles	0.25–0.27	0.34–0.35	ND	ND	40.5 –43.6	40.5 –43.6
Country Crisp	1.70–1.79	1.97–2.08	ND	< .5	17.5 –18.2	21.3 –22.0
Fortified Oat Flakes	0.20–0.24	0.20–0.32	ND	< .5	17.5 –17.7	18.2 –18.4
Frosted Rice Krinkles	0.25–0.28	0.41–0.46	ND	ND	40.0 –43.5	40.0 –43.5
Fruity Pebbles	0.21–0.23	0.33–0.36	ND	ND	41.3 –41.8	41.3 –41.8
Grape Nuts	0.74–0.77	1.38–1.41	ND	4.82–4.98	ND	7.01– 7.11
Grape Nuts Flakes	0.28–0.35	0.70–0.85	ND	4.09–4.93	6.83– 7.72	11.9 –13.7
Honey Combs	0.12–0.14	0.10–0.12	ND	ND	35.7 –39.0	35.7 –39.0
Post Toasties	1.17–1.19	1.40–1.45	ND	ND	2.59– 2.92	5.23– 5.49
Raisin Bran	6.40–7.62	6.22–7.41	ND	0.96–1.66	14.4 –15.4	28.0 –32.1
Super Sugar Crisp	2.20–2.40	4.49–4.93	ND	2.37–3.02	35.0 –36.6	44.9 –45.8

NOTE: Reprinted, with permission, from Betty Li and P. J. Schuhmann, *Journal of Food Science*, Vol. 45 (1980). The detection limit was 0.01 percent for fructose and glucose and 0.1 percent for lactose, maltose, and sucrose.
[a]ND = Not detectable.

PRODUCT	FRUCTOSE	GLUCOSE	LACTOSE	MALTOSE	SUCROSE	TOTAL SUGAR
Buckwheats	0.77–0.86	0.66–0.90	ND[a]	0.1 –0.4	9.56–11.4	11.0 –13.0
Cheerios	0.06–0.14	ND	ND	ND	2.58– 3.48	2.58– 3.48
Cocoa Puffs	0.10–0.16	1.65–1.89	ND	1.01–1.22	31.0 –32.1	34.0 –35.0
Count Chocula	0.13–0.41	3.01–4.88	0.15–0.32	ND	33.2 –37.3	36.5 –42.2
Crazy Cow, Chocolate	0.11–0.34	2.05–2.46	0.81–0.84	0.28–0.62	41.0 –43.7	43.9 –46.6
Crazy Cow, Strawberry	0.10–0.15	1.79–2.19	ND	< .5	36.1 –40.6	37.9 –42.6
Frankenberry	0.36–0.42	3.94–4.42	0.26–0.29	1.16–1.42	37.7 –38.9	43.7 –45.2
Golden Grahams	0.91–0.93	1.14–1.20	ND	ND	26.6 –28.2	28.7 –30.4
Kix	0.25–0.69	0.14–0.53	ND	ND	3.06– 4.83	3.06– 6.05
Lucky Charms	0.46–0.82	3.98–5.89	0.21–0.47	0.22–0.32	34.1 –37.4	38.5 –44.1
Total	0.69–0.90	0.44–0.62	ND	ND	5.54– 6.88	6.67– 8.16
	0.80–0.89	0.54–0.66	ND	ND	6.99– 7.58	8.48– 9.13
Trix	0.12–0.17	1.63–2.11	ND	0.57–1.06	28.5 –37.2	30.8 –40.5
Wheaties	0.60–0.86	0.36–0.58	ND	ND	6.70– 7.52	7.98– 8.48

NOTE: Reprinted, with permission, from Betty Li and P. J. Schuhmann, *Journal of Food Science,* Vol. 45 (1980). The detection limit was 0.01 percent for fructose and glucose and 0.1 percent for lactose, maltose, and sucrose.
[a]ND = Not detectable.

One way to study causal effects is with a challenge study. Two investigators have carried out such experiments. The National Institutes of Health researchers conducted studies with twenty-one children whose families had responded to an advertisement seeking children with adverse behavior patterns that supposedly worsened following sugar ingestion. The children received challenges of sucrose, glucose, or a sweet-tasting placebo.[42]

By adding saccharin to all three challenges, having the tests at least two days apart, and administering the substances as a lemon-flavored ice slurry, a double-blind study was maintained. This study found none of the behavioral changes that had been observed by the mothers. Furthermore, children with no psychiatric diagnosis as well as those with one or more psychiatric diagnoses were found to be significantly less active on sugar.

In contrast, at Children's Hospital in Washington, D.C., investigators gave regular orange juice or juice sweetened with sucrose or fructose to thirteen emotionally ill children.[43] Compared to the control group, the children who received sugar showed an increase in total activity.

CAFFEINE AND KIDS

Cola drinks are popular among youngsters. How much does their caffeine affect the brainpower of kids?

A study was done in which thirty high-caffeine consumers were found among eight hundred schoolchildren. The high-caffeine consumers were matched against children (controls) who reported low caffeine consumption.

High consumers were more likely than low consumers to be rated hyperactive by their teachers, and one-third of the high caffeine-consuming group—nine out of thirty—met the criterion for clinical hyperactivity based on their teacher rating scale scores.

Nineteen of the high-caffeine group and nineteen of the matched low consumers agreed to participate in a double-blind placebo controlled-challenge study, in which they received 10 milligrams of caffeine or placebo each day for two weeks. On caffeine, the low-caffeine consumers were rated as more emotional, inattentive, and restless by their parents, while high-caffeine consumers were not rated as significantly changed.

The differences between low and high consumers could not be attributed to tolerance, withdrawal, or subject selection and thus suggest a possible physiological basis in children for dietary caffeine preference. Moreover, the study points out the importance of challenge studies. The initial data would have indicated that the caffeine caused the hyperactivity. Instead, the challenge data indicated that hyperactive children might selectively ingest caffeine, quite the contrary finding.[44]

Caffeine may serve to calm the hyperactive, a paradoxical phenomenon also found when stimulant drugs are given to hyperactive children to sedate them.

Doris L. Pertz, a learning disabilities teacher and consultant in the Caldwell–West Caldwell (New Jersey) public schools, and Lillian Putnam, director of the reading clinic at the Caldwell public schools and a professor at Kean College of New Jersey in Union, pointed out that eating a nutritious breakfast results in improved student attention in late-morning task performance:

> In early life, caloric deficits lead to reduction of activity—less play with peers, less verbalizing and less sensory stimulation. Because of this, these children enter school with minimal readiness for learning. A low level of sensory stimulation in preschool years and poor attention in the school-age child are associated with later manifestations of intellectual deficit.[45]

Poor nutrition also increases absenteeism because it reduces the body's capacity to resist disease and infections.

Anemia caused by an iron-deficient diet also affects learning. A child's brain uses about half of the oxygen supply carried in the blood. Iron-deficient blood does not carry a normal oxygen load. There is some thought that a low blood-oxygen level due to iron deficiency may contribute to reading disability.[46]

In addition, as pointed out in the toxicology and allergy chapters, a child who is suffering an adverse reaction to foods can have reduced attention to the learning task.

Pertz and Putnam suggest:

• Teachers should work with parents and school authorities to remove candy, soft drinks, and caffeine beverages from vending machines and school cafeterias. These should be replaced with fruits, nuts, milk, and fruit drinks.

• Teachers should discourage fund-raising projects that rely on the sale of candy. Sales can emphasize nuts, dried fruits, and nonedible items.[47]

DIET AND SCHOOL PERFORMANCE

Can you give children a healthy, well-balanced diet that is low in food additives and sugar and see a difference in their intellectual performance?

A diet policy in 803 New York City schools was changed over a period of four years. The amount of sugary foods and synthetically colored and flavored foods as well as foods preserved with BHA and BHT was lowered over that four-year period.

The impact of a low-additive and sugar-reduced diet on academic performance in these schools was studied by Stephen J. Schoenthaler, Ph.D., Walter Doraz, Ph.D., and James Wakefield, Jr., Ph.D. They reported that the change in food policy was followed by a 15.7 percent increase in mean academic percentile, ranking above the rest of the nation's schools that used the same standardized tests. Prior to the 15.7-percent gain, the standard deviation of the annual change in national percentile ratings had been less than 1 percent. Each school's academic performance ranking was negatively correlated with the percent of children who ate school food before the diet policy changes. However, after the menu changes, the percent of students who ate school lunches and breakfasts within each school became positively correlated with that school's rate of gain. Before the diet change, very little change had occurred in mean academic percentile rank for the 803 schools.[48]

Dr. Schoenthaler and his colleagues say one question remains unanswered: "Was the change in performance due to the combination of restriction food additives, sucrose, and fat or to an unidentified factor which is correlated with all three, such as malnutrition?"[49]

The researchers said that lay people might be tempted to conclude that sugar and food additives directly caused the poor grades, with the fat being the least important factor. Most nutritionists, on the other hand, would assume that a reduction in malnutrition—rather than a reduction in sugar, fats, and food additives—is probably the primary cause of the improved academic performance, for three reasons:

1. A common factor exists in foods that contain high levels of fats, sucrose, and food additives. They tend to be low in the ratio of essential nutrients to calories. Foods that are laden with synthetic food colors and flavors tend to be the more processed foods that, in turn, have lost a substantial portion of their nutritional value in processing. Pure sucrose, by definition, contains no nutrient other than four calories per gram. Fat contains a few nutrients but has even more calories per gram—9 grams. When the consumption of empty calories (sucrose, fats, and processed foods) decreases, children normally eat other foods that contain a higher ratio of nutrients to calories. The uptake in foods that are more nutritious should lower any malnutrition that existed.

2. A substantial body of research supports the link between malnutrition and academic behavior in controlled laboratory studies.

3. The available data published in major journals that directly implicate food additives and sucrose consistently point to negative findings in general or else positive findings in a very select population.

Dr. Schoenthaler and his colleagues conclude:

> Improvements in academic performance by comparison with other U.S. schools during the same time period appear to be due to the diet policies which restricted fats, sucrose and food additives. The cause will remain unverified without further research, but malnutrition may be the predominate cause since all students have the potential of being malnourished. Although malnutrition appears to be the most likely theoretical explanation for most of the improvements, selected children have improved due to restrictions of food additives and sucrose which cause "allergy" symptoms.[50]

GENERAL RULES OF A HEALTHY DIET FOR CHILDREN TODAY

Balance and moderation are the best rules to follow when it comes to diets for adults or for children. The following are the general regulations for a healthy diet for children, based on a compilation of sources from government and health organizations:[51]

- **Total fat** intake should be approximately 30 percent of calories, with 10 percent or less from saturated fat, about 10 percent from monounsaturated fat, and less than 10 percent from polyunsaturated fat. The emphasis should be on reduction of total fat and, especially, saturated fat rather than an increase in polyunsaturated fat.

- **Daily cholesterol** intake should be approximately 100 milligrams of cholesterol per 1,000 calories, not to exceed 300 milligrams. This allows for differences in caloric intake in various age groups.

- **Protein** should be about 15 percent of calories, derived from various sources.

- **Carbohydrate** calories should be derived primarily from complex carbohydrate sources to provide necessary vitamins and minerals. Thus, the total calories from carbohydrates would be about 55 percent.

- **Salt** intake should be reduced. On the whole, the American diet contains too much salt, so keep the salt shaker out of reach. High blood pressure in children does occur, and it is believed that the child who is in the ninetieth percentile for blood pressure will go on to develop high blood pressure by the age of thirty-five or forty years.

Menu choices for children that fit the aforementioned criteria:

MEAL	FOOD	SERVING SIZE
Breakfast	**Protein**	
	egg or	1
	peanut butter or	1 ounce
	cheese	1 ounce
	Fat	
	margarine or	
	butter	1 pat
	Carbohydrate	
	bread or	1 to 2 slices
	cereal	½ to 1 cup
	Calcium	
	milk or	1 cup
	yogurt	1 cup

TABLE—*continued*

MEAL	FOOD	SERVING SIZE
	Fruit	
	orange or	1
	fruit juice or	1 cup
	apple	1
Lunch	**Protein**	
	chicken or	3 ounces
	tuna or	3 ounces
	cheese	3 ounces
	Carbohydrate	
	bread or	1 slice
	pasta	1 cup
	Fat	
	butter or	1 pat
	mayonnaise	1 tablespoon
	Vegetable	
	lettuce and/or	several leaves
	carrot sticks or	4
	celery	2
	Fruit	
	apple or	1
	orange or	1
	dried apricots	½ cup
	Calcium	
	milk or	1 cup
	yogurt	1 cup
Dinner	**Protein**	
	broiled or baked fish, poultry, or beef;	4 to 6 ounces
	or legumes	1 cup cooked
	Carbohydrate	
	pasta or	¾ cup cooked
	bread or	1 to 2 slices
	rice	¾ cup cooked
	Vegetables	
	green salad or	small plate
	carrots or peas or	
	broccoli or spinach	¾ cup cooked
	Fat	
	butter or	1 pat
	margarine or	1 pat
	mayonnaise or	2 tablespoons
	salad dressing	2 tablespoons

TABLE—*continued*

MEAL	FOOD	SERVING SIZE
	Calcium	
	milk or	1 glass
	ice cream or	1 scoop
	frozen yogurt	1 scoop
	Fruit	
	apple or orange or	1
	grapes or	1 bunch
	fruit cup or	1 cup
	fruit juice	6 ounces
	Snacks	
	Any fruit or juice or	1 piece or 1 cup
	nuts or	$\frac{1}{3}$ cup
	popcorn or	2 cups popped
	whole-wheat crackers or	4
	fruit pops	1

As a parent, one of the most important gifts you can give your child is a wise way of eating. It will help his brain and body develop to their full potential and will probably make him easier to live with.

⚔ 10 ⚔

Maintaining and Improving Adult Brain Power Through Food

You have spent your life, thus far, with certain eating and living habits, some good and some bad. You have a measure of control over your habits—the diet you eat and the amount of exercise you get and whether you smoke cigarettes or drink alcoholic beverages. A number of the physical and mental changes you experience from day to day are influenced by your habits. Others result directly from the wear and tear of the passing years.

How many of the changes we associate with age are due to the passing of years and how many are the result of years of passing up the right foods?

Almost all experts agree that the foods we select are a big factor in maintaining the health of our brains and bodies, but there is much yet to be learned about the nutritional needs of specific ages. The RDA's are based on healthy young males, while it is now accepted that the nutritional needs of a twenty year old, a fifty year old, and a seventy year old are very different.

The RDA for calcium is a prime example of the limitation of extrapolating recommendations from data collected on a younger population. Age-related decreases in bone mass actually begin around the age of twenty years in both men and women, progressing at a rate of 6 to 10 percent per year. Bone loss produces age-dependent susceptibility to fractures. The level of dietary calcium currently recommended for adults is 800 milligrams per day, but postmenopausal women are now believed to need a calcium intake as high as 1,500 milligrams per day to help prevent bone loss.

Kidney and liver functions may decline 20 to 30 percent between the

189

ages of fifty years and ninety years. Both organs are involved in clearing drugs and foods from the body. This has been shown in the amount of time it takes to clear the drug diazepam (the muscle relaxant Valium) from the body after ingestion. On the average, it takes a fifty year old fifty-five hours and an eighty year old as long as ninety hours to clear the drug.

One change that occurs as the years pass is the rate at which your body uses energy while at rest—the basal metabolism rate—which slows down as the total amount of lean body tissue decreases and the amount of total body fat increases.

But how much of the slowed metabolism is due to aging and how much is due to too much fat and sugar in the diet? How much do stress or exercise affect how you process food?

Edward Schneider, M.D., of the National Institutes of Health and his colleagues point out that on the one hand, a cut in calories has been recommended for us as we grow older, to adjust for our slowed metabo-

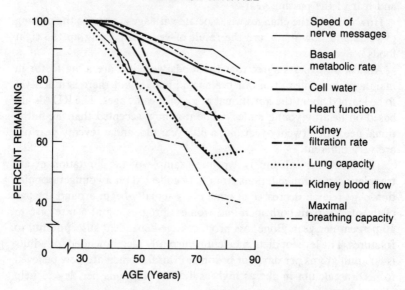

REDUCTION IN PHYSIOLOGICAL FUNCTION WITH AGE

Graph adapted from Strohler, B. L., Origin of the effects of time and high-energy radiation on living systems. Quarterly Review Biology. 34: (2), 117-142 (1959)

lism and our decrease in physical activity. The slower metabolism results in a reduction in lean body mass. On the other hand, an increased intake of calcium has been recommended for older women, to counter the age-associated decline in bone mass. The recommended changes in intake are based on the assumption that the age-related declines in muscle and activity levels are normal and harmless, but that the decline in bone mass is abnormal. However, researchers such as Dr. Schneider now suggest that many of the age-related disabilities of the brain and body might be decreased if lean body mass and physical activity were maintained rather than diminished in older persons.[1]

Jeff Blumberg, Ph.D., assistant director of the Tufts Center on Nutrition and the Aging, says,

> We're questioning the basic assumption that older people require smaller amounts of nutrients because their bodies are slowing down and because they're less active. While their calorie requirements may be diminished because they are less active, their nutrient requirements are the same or may be even greater than they were. Perhaps if elderly people get more of certain nutrients, the aging process may slow down.[2]

One of the nutrients that older people may need to increase is protein. Lean body mass declines with age, it is believed, because of changes in protein absorption or metabolism or both.[3] Therefore, older people may need more protein, not only for lean body mass but because their brain's neurotransmitters are made from protein bases. For example, the amino acid serine, a building block of protein, is a base material for choline which, in turn, is made into acetylcholine in the body. Acetylcholine is a neurotransmitter that sends messages between brain cells and is involved in memory.

As we grow older, most of us begin to have problems with our memories: Where did I put those keys? What is her name? Why did I open the refrigerator door? In fact, such problems are so common that they are called "benign senile forgetfulness." (Then, of course, there is the devastating brain degenerative disease that affects more than two-million Americans and their families—Alzheimer's—in which the loss of memory is severe.)

What happens to the brain and its memory function as we age, and what part does nutrition play?

Remember that old belief that fish is brain food? There may be some truth to it, because fish contains high levels of choline, as do meat and eggs. Choline is made from food in the body, taken from the digestive tract by the blood and carried to the brain where it becomes acetylcholine.

As we age, the capability of transferring information from one cell to another or to a target organ is markedly reduced. In part, this is due to the amount of acetylcholine and in part to the ability to use what is there. An enzyme used to produce acetylcholine is *N-acetyltransferase.* Interestingly, it has been discovered that stress depresses the amount of acetyltransferase. We've all experienced difficulty when trying to think under stress—blame your acetyltransferase.

Raymond Bartus, Ph.D., one of the nation's foremost experts on memory and director of the Geriatric Research Discovery Program of the Department of Central Nervous System Research, Lederle Laboratories, Pearl River, New York, says one of the most consistent neurochemical findings is the reduced activity of choline acetyltransferase in the aged human brain and its markedly reduced activity in the brains of Alzheimer's victims.

Choline, possibly because nature recognized its importance, is the only neurotransmitter that has been found that can be made from another dietary component besides protein. The amino acid *serine,* derived from protein, is a basic material for choline, but so is *lecithin,* which is found in large amounts in eggs. In addition to the lack of serine and lecithin in the diet, lack of sufficient B_{12} and folic acid can also affect the formation of the brain neurotransmitter acetylcholine. Do elderly persons hampered by the lack of money to buy protein foods become deficient in choline? If so, they would lack acetylcholine to charge their brain cells and thus would probably exhibit the memory deficits so common even in "normal" aging.

There has been an effort to increase the building blocks of acetylcholine by increasing lecithin, the normal source of choline in the diet. This has been disappointing so far. Dairy products and meats contain significant amounts of lecithin. The Thomas J. Lipton company has produced a lecithin-enriched chicken noodle soup as a method of supplying large amounts of this chemical to the brain. Lipton is scheduled to put the soup on the market in 1988 without any medical claims for the product, just calling it "chicken soup with lecithin." The purified lecithin, which is more concentrated than that sold in health food stores, raises blood levels of choline, which, in turn, may aid memory. According to Lederle's Dr. Bartus, animal studies suggest that increasing lecithin in the diet may prevent, not cure, memory deficits.

As of this writing, a combination of lecithin and *piracetam,* a synthetic compound derived from alcohol, seems to affect brain energy and facilitate performance on measures of learning and retention in brain-injured and aged rates. It also appears to protect against impairment caused by lack of oxygen in animals. Piracetam is being tested on brain-injured children but seems to work better when combined with lecithin than either substance works alone. Preliminary studies in five geriatric centers suggest that some patients may respond positively to this treatment.

While the exact role and requirement of choline in the diet remains unknown, the brain is unable to make choline itself. It must be derived from the diet or from choline manufactured by the liver.[4] As far back as the September 8, 1977, issue of the *New England Journal of Medicine,* researchers from MIT reported choline supplementation could relieve the involuntary facial twitching of persons suffering from tardive dyskinesia, a brain ailment common in long-time antipychotic drug users.

The concept that the impairment of the brain's system for using choline in certain diseases and in old age may be prevented or minimized by adding choline-base materials to the diet is certainly worth pursuing. Researchers agree that the importance of adequate amounts of choline or lecithin in the diet should not be minimized and that the amount probably varies greatly with age, disease, and the composition of other foods in the diet.

Robert Butler, M.D., a leading expert on aging and former director of the National Institute on Aging, points out in the text *Nutrition in the 1980s:*

> There is some evidence that behavior can be modified by dietary supplementation with such substances as choline, tryptophan and tyrosine. These substances increase the brain concentrations of the neurotransmitters acetylcholine, serotonin and dopamine.
>
> Perhaps research regarding the nutritional contribution to central nervous system neurotransmitter function will help in the treatment of senile dementia. This is one of the most feared afflictions of later life. It is a heavy emotional and economic drain on families and society, and it costs the United States billions of dollars for care in nursing facilities.
>
> There are also nutritional deficiencies that account for treatable forms

of "senility"—treatable if diagnosed. For example, older persons with pernicious anemia may appear confused and forgetful. A thorough diagnostic work up will reveal the basis for the apparent senility, and proper management may reverse the symptoms.

It is entirely possible that chronic marginal deficiencies in nutrition contribute much more than we now recognize to the problem of senility. There is evidence of the decline with age in dopamine and choline acetylase activity in the brains of experimental animals. Patients with senile dementia of the Alzheimer type are reported to have diminished levels of choline acetyltransferase and choline acetylase. The possibility that a dietary source of choline can be used to treat senile dementia of the Alzheimer's type has been suggested but not established.[5]

Dr. Butler expressed the hope that attempts to relate dietary factors to senile dementia and other chronic diseases will continue.

Another way that diet can affect memory was reported in 1987. James F. Flood, Ph.D., of the Psychobiology Research Laboratory at the Geriatric Research Center of the Veterans Administration Medical Center in Sepulveda, California, and his colleagues, subjected groups of mice to different feeding routines while the mice were taught how to run a maze.[6] One of the basic needs of even the most primitive organism is to find food. The advantage to the animal of maintaining a vivid memory of a successful hunt is obvious. The researchers reasoned that feeding animals right after a training session would enhance the animal's memories. The ability to remember the right route was best in those animals that ate voraciously after learning. The memory/eating connection was found to be linked to the stomach neurotransmitter cholecystokinin (CCK), which is secreted during eating and is one of several neurotransmitters that carry messages to your brain to stop eating. CCK acts on the vagus nerve, which connects your stomach to your brain. When the vagus nerve was severed in the animal experiments, the memory effect of the after-learning meal was lost.

Dr. Flood speculates that the association of eating with memory may have given wild animals a survival advantage—eating caused the release of CCK, which in turn telegraphed the message along the vagus nerve to the brain. The enhanced memory of the animal, therefore, helped it to survive by filing away the successful food-hunting strategy.

So, the next time you have something to remember, study it and then eat a good meal that releases your CCK. Since the amino acids phenylalanine and tryptophan are reported to increase the amount of CCK released, that meal could include milk (high in phenylalanine) and nuts, rice, or seeds (all high in tryptophan).

Two other dietary substances are also being intensively studied as factors in the decline of brain function we associate with aging: fat and sugar.

THE DESTRUCTIVE SINGLES

Chemical compounds consist of two or more elements that are bound together by a chemical bond. The bonding involves negatively charged parts of the elements called electrons. The arrangement of the electrons determines the stability of the compounds. A stable compound has electrons that are in pairs, somewhat like a buddy system. On the other hand, if an electron does not have a partner, it can be come very reactive and unstable. It will seek out another electron to pair up with in order to return to a stable state. A compound or element with an unpaired electron is called a "free radical."

Like the "other woman" in an affair, a free radical will seek out and grab an electron from a stable compound. This action, in turn, can create a new free radical. A chain reaction takes place that continues until the unpaired electron can pair up with another unpaired electron or is deactivated by an antioxidant, scavenger cell, or enzyme.

Free radicals are formed daily though normal body processes. In addition, certain environmental pollutants can react within the body to cause the generation of free radicals. These include free radicals formed by radiation, air pollution, cigarette smoke, and herbicides. Although free radicals are highly reactive, unstable species that are generated in the body, they have the potential to cause severe damage to cell structures.

Free radicals have been associated with oxidation of body fat (rancidity), which causes damage in cell membranes and can produce cell death. Free radicals have also been associated with damage to the nucleus of cells, including DNA breakage, which can potentially induce cancer, destruction of the cells that line the blood vessels in vital organs, and inflammation in arthritic joints. Free radicals have been tagged as hasteners of the aging process and as factors in lung injury as well as in the brain damage that results in senility. Free radicals are also suspects in the cause of Alzheimer's disease.[7]

Vitamin C, vitamin E, and beta carotene in your diet help protect your body and brain against free radicals because they prevent oxidation.

Scientists have known for some time that another natural antioxidant exists that can be found in onions, garlic, peppers, soybeans, and many green leafy plants.

Professor Dan Pratt of Purdue University's foods and nutrition department is testing plant compounds for their antioxidant properties. Oxidation is a problem for foods such as meat, oil, salad dressing, shortening, nuts, butter, cereal, and many novelty and commercial foods.

Says Dr. Pratt, "We knew, for example, that if you take two beakers of stew meat, one with vegetables and one without, that spoilage will occur first in the one without the vegetables. But few researchers focused on determining what within the plants was doing the work."[8]

Dr. Pratt and his research team have tested such plants as avocados, soybeans, and more exotic plants like chia, a desert plant with a small seed that Indians used to eat for energy.

"We found that chia seed is the best one we've tried," Dr. Pratt says. "In a lot of cases, it's not the edible part of the plant that is high in antioxidants. For example, the seed of the pepper is much higher in antioxidants than the pepper pod; the skin of the potato has more than the inside of the potato."[9]

This oxidation process may play a part in schizophrenia as well as senility. Abraham Hoffer, M.D., suggested thirty years ago that oxidative stress was a factor in schizophrenia. He proposed that some neurotransmitters could become irreversibly oxidized in the body and damage brain tissues.

Newer evidence lends support to Dr. Hoffer's theory that schizophrenia may involve brain tissue damage from oxidized neurotransmitter derivatives.[10]

A number of researchers now believe that including antioxidants in your diet can prevent or slow brain cell damage from oxidized fat.

SUGAR AND AGING

Sugar is another element in our diets that is a candidate for being an aging factor. Anthony Cerami, Ph.D., who heads the Rockefeller University's Laboratory of Medical Biochemistry, believes that many of the breakdowns associated with age proceed from a single, fundamental chemical reaction between glucose and the proteins that comprise the body's metabolic machinery and structural framework.

"Until recently, glucose was generally considered a stable and innocuous molecule serving as a central source for energy. Scientists have since learned that it not only plays a part in metabolism—the body's use of energy—but also that this abundant and ubiquitous sugar is not always benign,"[11] says Dr. Cerami.

Most biological activities are triggered by chemical catalysts called enzymes. Glucose, however, has the ability to react with proteins and with nucleic acids (the genetic material of cells) just by being next to them, a process called *nonenzymatic glycosylation.*

"A lot of complicated chemistry goes on," says Dr. Cerami, "and if the reaction is permitted to continue, eventually it produces a brownish-yellow pigment that can bind two molecules together."[12]

In other words, blood sugar can jumble protein and tangle molecules, leaving undisposed garbage in the cell.

Dr. Cerami has named the resulting pigments "AGE," for advanced glycosylated end-products. The manufacture of these sugar-modified proteins is independent of the amount of sugar we consume. The body can produce glucose from starch and other foodstuffs, so the formation of AGE is a continuous, life-long process whenever blood glucose is permitted to react with proteins.

One familiar manifestation of AGE is the browning of food. The skin of a roasted chicken turns brown because the dehydration that occurs during cooking accelerates the formation of AGE. The same thing happens when bread is toasted. The effects of AGE over time can be observed simply by comparing the brown, hard, dried apricots from a health food store with the artificially preserved supermarket variety, which are bright orange and soft. Pathologists have observed that the bones of older people are browner than the bones of younger people. "Like untreated apricots," says Dr. Cerami, "we're browning all the time."

AGE does more than just discolor tissue. As Dr. Cerami explains, "AGE acts as a chemical glue to attach molecules to one another, forming what we call a cross-link. That is why overcooked meat is so difficult to slice and chew. You are literally sawing through cross-linked proteins with your knife and grinding them down with your teeth."[13]

Dr. Ceramin maintains that these same glucose-derived cross-links have been traced to many physical manifestations of old age. While eating browned chicken and toast may not "age" you, understanding the process of why these foods turn brown may go far in helping scientists understand the process of human aging and thus how to slow it down.

STRESS AND DIGESTION

Can stress—from the little aggravations of everyday living such as traffic jams to the big stressors such as loss of job or loved one—contribute to these aging changes in fat and sugar? Here the pieces of the puzzle fit together nicely.

Stress affects many body processes and the digestive and central nervous systems are no exception. Researchers have found that if the stress is short-lived, the changes in stress hormone levels will be transient and unlikely to induce a breakdown response. If, on the other hand, the stress is intense or applied for an extended period of time, changes in the hormonal system can lead to a breakdown of body substances, such as proteins. Another factor is that not all persons react equally to the same stress.

Although precise signals that initiate the speedup of metabolism under stress are unknown, several lines of evidence point to the role of the brain. A wide variety of stresses stimulate the hypothalamus, the area of the brain involved in eating behavior and in sending commands to the pituitary gland to relay a message to the adrenal glands to release stress hormones. The stress hormones are then carried in the blood and transmit a return message to the brain to release its own stress neurotransmitters. This system makes sense. Your adrenals prepare your body to fight or flee by making your heart beat faster and your muscles tense up, and then your brain decides whether to stand and fight or to beat a hasty retreat with your well-prepared body.

These circulating stress chemicals also affect sugar and fat metabolism. They interfere with energy storage and protein metabolism. So you see how stress can add its damage to those caused by free radicals and AGE.

COMBATING STRESS, FREE RADICALS, AND AGE

In addition to eating plenty of natural antioxidants in such foods as carrots, lettuce, and oranges, cutting down on fat and sugar in your diet, and easing stress in your life, what else can you do? Exercise!

Researchers at the University of Rochester School of Medicine reported at a 1986 Society for Neuroscience meeting that a prolonged high-fat, high-sugar diet exerts a chronic effect on the part of the brain related to the endocrine system, but that this effect can be retarded by moderate exercise.[14] The affected brain region, the hypothalamus, is responsible for the production of the hormone vasopressin, which affects various heart, blood vessel, kidney, metabolic, behavioral, and immunologic functions. Vasopressin plays a part in memory and stress. These findings may be relevant to aging, since excess fat and high sugar consumption may worsen the changes that normally occur in the vasopressin system during aging.

Oxytocin is another pituitary hormone associated with the autonomic nervous system that controls heartbeat, breathing, and other automatic functions. It is also involved in the production of breast milk, uterine contractions, maternal behavior, and immunity.

The hormonal and autonomic nervous systems are major routes by which your brain communicates with the rest of your body. Both vasopressin and oxytocin may play a part in stress-induced eating and in cravings for carbohydrates. Some researchers now think that vasopressin may play a role in binge eating. Others have shown that vasopressin is affected by diets deficient in certain nutrients and that it may play an important function in the metabolic reaction to stress. Oxytocin, on the other hand, circulates in the blood and promotes the growth of fat cells, while brain oxytocin has been related to certain types of obesity. From these findings, it seems that a prolonged high-fat, high-sugar diet would hinder vasopressin and oxytocin functioning and that moderate exercise might protect against this perturbation.

Animal experiments found that prolonged high-fat, high-sugar diets substantially depleted the vasopressin content of the areas related to the neuroendocrine system, which, in turn, promoted an apparent further sugar intake. Moderate exercise was shown to retard this vasopressin activity and thereby reduce cravings for sugar.

The investigators also found that high-fat, high-sugar intake associated with obesity caused an increase in the amount of oxytocin in the blood. Because oxytocin enhances fat cell growth, the increased levels of oxytocin that accompany obesity may promote further weight gain. Exercise had no effect on oxytocin in the blood, but it did substantially increase the oxytocin content of an area of the brain involved in blood pressure regulation.

Exercise can also help your brain control your appetite. In a study reported in journal *Metabolism* in 1985, Dr. R. Wood and F. Pi-Sunyer analyzed the effect of increased physical activity on the voluntary intake of lean women.[15] They found that exercise burns up excess calories, promotes weight loss in the obese, and helps people control their desire to eat.

The study involved both obese and lean women who normally did not exercise. The women were offered excessive amounts of food daily for three nineteen-day periods. During each period, a different level of activity was required—sedentary, mild, and then moderate. The women's voluntary food intake was monitored and records were kept of both daily food intake and prescribed exercise on a treadmill.

The caloric data showed that exercise had not significantly inhibited food intake in either the obese or the lean women. At no time was intake during exercise less than during the sedentary periods.

These data suggest that energy stores in the body may regulate eating behavior. As activity increased, the obese women in the study did not eat more food. Instead, they lost weight by using up stored fat. In contrast, the lean women maintained their weight by eating more.

The researchers summarized that to maintain weight, energy output must still equal energy intake. When output exceeds intake, one loses weight. When output is lower, one gains weight and the difference is stored as fat.

When you cut back on food intake, your body's natural tendency is to conserve energy, leading to as much as a 15- to 30-percent decrease in basal metabolic rate.[16]

Fortunately, physical activity counteracts this diet-related decrease in metabolism, as evidenced by another recent study. Obese people on very low calorie diets had a gradual reduction in metabolic rate over a two-week period. But when they started to exercise for twenty to thirty minutes a day, their rates returned to normal within three or four days. At the end of two weeks, the rates were even higher. On the other hand, obese individuals who were on the same diet for four weeks but who did not exercise showed nearly a 20-percent reduction in basal metabolic rate.[17]

You know that old joke about the old man who exclaimed, "If I had known I was going to live so long, I would have taken better care of myself!"? Well, we *are* living longer, but we also want to live better—that is, we want to keep our brains and bodies in the best shape possible. As far as protecting your brain is concerned, you can't do anything about your heredity, but you can do something about your diet.

THE GOLDEN RULES OF HEALTHY EATING

Variety and moderation. Reduce or moderate your fat (especially animal and other saturated fats), cholesterol, and salt intake and eat more whole grains, vegetables, and fruits. If food choices are limited because of availability, preferences, and abnormal digestion or metabolism, seek expert help. Your physician or local hospital dietician may be able to advise you.

Keep up with your protein. Amino acids, from which the brain's neuro-transmitters are made, come from protein in the diet, as pointed out many times in this book. There is a lot of emphasis in the lay and medical literature on complex carbohydrates, but the older you get, the more protein you may need. In fact, the RDA of protein is 56 grams for adult men and 45 grams for women, but some people may need as much as 80 to 90 grams of protein per day, depending on their physical condition. For others with kidney or liver problems, protein in their diet may need to be reduced. Check with your physician.

Go easy on the sugar. As we get older, our tolerance for sugar in the blood may become less. When you can, take your sugar in the form of fruit (see chapter 3).

Eat some of your vegetables and fruits raw. If your digestive apparatus permits, eat as much as half of your fruits and vegetables raw. Processing causes many fruits and vegetables to lose some of their vitamins. Freezing kills the vitamin E, for example, and storage depletes the vitamin C in orange juice. Raw foods may be more filling and satisfying than highly processed foods, and the fiber aids elimination.

Be sure you get enough of the B vitamins. The B vitamins are vital to the nerves and brain. As we get older, we may have more trouble absorbing these vitamins. (See chapter 3 for foods that are high in B vitamins.) You may need B_{12} or B_6 by injection because you are not absorbing enough by mouth. Ask your physician.

Be sure you get enough vitamins A, C, and E. These antioxidant vitamins can help protect your cells against the wear and tear that occurs with age. (See chapter 3 for foods that are rich in these vitamins.) It is best to get vitamin A from beta carotene, vitamin A's precursor in vegetables (see page 36). It also is wise to obtain vitamins C and E from food, but supplementary vitamins C and E can't hurt and they may help significantly.

Don't succumb to the single-eater syndrome. Many people in our society live alone. The tendency for single eaters is to not fuss with meals and to gulp down whatever is handy in the refrigerator or on the shelf. Instead, make sure your meals are attractive and balanced. You need protein, fresh fruits and vegetables, and carbohydrates even if you dine alone. Treat yourself as you would a guest. An attractively set table with flowers or other decorations can help nourish your brain as well as your body.

Taste and smell sensitivity may need a boost. If you find that your food tastes too bland, use more herbs and spices. Tart foods may enhance flavors. Orange juice, lemonade, vinegar, and lemon juice used as seasonings may help. Many foods taste better if they are either cold or at room temperature. Try new taste treats. There are a lot of ethnic foods, and if they are novel to you, that may spark your taste and capture your interest. If you find you have a problem with lack of ability to taste or smell, consult your physician. You may benefit from a zinc supplement.

Opt for low-fat treats. Junkets, puddings, or shakes made with skim milk; angel food cake; popsicles; sherbet; gelatin ice; hard and jelly candies; and no-salt pretzels are good choices for low-fat treats.

Take a walk. Numerous studies have shown that exercise aids metabolism and is good not only for the body but also for the brain. Walking is probably the most beneficial since it doesn't stress the joints or injure the shoulders or neck, as many popular exercises may do. If you do nothing more than park the car a little farther from the store than you usually do and walk that extra distance, you will benefit. Walking in place can be fun if you do it to the beat of your favorite music.

Don't bring your troubles to the table. You may be having work or family problems, but make it an unbreakable rule to leave them out of the dining area. Stress inhibits digestion and keeps you from obtaining the proper nourishment for your brain.

Use your brain to motivate yourself. Anyone over age thirty-five usually has special physical conditions that may warrant more of some things in the diet and less of others. By now, you've read this book and probably many other books and articles on nutrition. You *know* what you should and should not eat. Make promises to yourself about how you are going to change your diet for the better. Write down those promises. Post them on your refrigerator. You may not keep all of them, but they may help you make some improvements. And before you eat something when you are not hungry or that you know is not good for you, ask yourself, Do I really want to eat this? Ask yourself five times. If the answer is still yes do it, but don't do it too often!

◁ 11 ▷

Hunger, Appetite, and Your Brain

W hy do you eat?
  Are you hungry?
  Have you eaten when you had no appetite, just to be sociable
or because it's time for a meal?

Do you continue to eat when you're no longer hungry?

What's the difference between hunger and appetite?

The answers to all of the above lie within your brain and the messages
it sends and receives from other parts of your body.

First of all, hunger is the *need* for food. Appetite is the *desire* for food.
You can have an appetite without being hungry, and you can be hungry
and not have an appetite, as in the case of anoretics who literally starve
themselves (see page 215).

While your hunger may be based more on your physical needs and
your appetite influenced more by culture and experience, both are regulated by your brain and both affect your brain function.

It was believed, at one time, that your stomach contractions and
"growling" informed your brain when you were hungry. We now know
that the message is much more complicated and involves a variety of
chemical signals to and from your brain that turn on and off your hunger.

As Albert Stunkard, M.D., professor of psychiatry at the University
of Pennsylvania and an expert in diet behavior, points out, most of us
have a greater problem not with starting to eat but with stopping.[1]

SATIETY CENTER

The search for the "stop-eating" control—the satiety center—in the
brain began around 1940, when researchers inserted electrodes in the
brains of rats and created various lesions. When a place in the center of

an area of the brain, the *ventromedial hypothalamus* (**VMH**), was destroyed, the rats ate excessively and became obese.[2] The VHM seemed to be the long-sought satiety center.

A similar condition of insatiable hunger occurs in human victims of Prader-Willis syndrome, a congenital defect of unknown origin in which a person is retarded and tremendously obese. These individuals are constantly preoccupied with food and will eat as long as food is available. They will steal food and gobble down garbage or pet food if meals are restricted. Researchers believe Prader-Willis victims never reach satiety.[3]

The hypothalamus is a tiny segment of nerve cells in the brain. It weighs less than four grams, but it provides a connecting link between your cerebral cortex (your "thinking" brain) and your pituitary gland. Although the pituitary gland has long been considered the "master gland," it is now known that it takes its orders from the hypothalamus, which sends it chemical instructions. Your hypothalamus regulates your energy through control of your appetite, sleep, body temperature, and water balance. This biologic computer in your brain is the switch panel of your complex and interrelated hormonal system. It governs your blood pressure and even takes part in the complex biochemical reactions that accompany your powerful emotions.

Since the hypothalamus is the control center for so many functions, it is easy to see how one of its duties—control of eating behavior—can be influenced by its other jobs, such as control over sexual excitement, mood, or temperature. If you are in a very hot dining room without air conditioning, for example, your appetite will certainly be dampened. And a starving person is more interested in finding food than in finding someone with whom to have a sexual encounter.

HUNGER CENTER

Scientists reasoned that if the VMH contained the satiety center, then perhaps there was another area of the hypothalamus that contained the hunger center. In 1951, researchers reported that rats who had a specific area of the hypothalamus destroyed would never eat again and would eventually die of starvation.[4] Three years later, Eliot Stellar, Ph.D., of the University of Pennsylvania's Department of Psychology, formally proposed that the center of the hypothalamus, the VMH, is the brain's satiety center and the side of the hypothalamus, the lateral hypothalamus

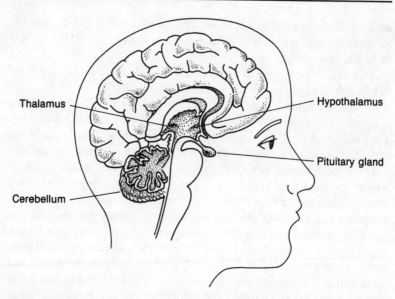

(LH), is its hunger center.[5] Although he acknowledged that there must be other factors involved, he maintained that these centers in the brain receive information through special sensory receptors in the hypothalamus that process the information and cause an action.

The hypothalamus, like any executive, must receive feedback from the field. It is generally agreed that those signals must be carried in the blood.[6]

The glucostatic theory of hunger says that the signal to stop eating comes from the level of sugar in the blood. Dr. Jean Mayer, president of Tufts University and an internationally known physiologist and nutritionist, concluded in 1952 that circulating sugar levels indicate the amount of immediately available or needed energy. Other substances such as fat or protein do not fit the picture because their concentration in the blood vary very little. Blood sugar, in contrast, increases quickly following eating and slowly decreases until the next meal.[7] Blood sugar is also known to be the primary energy source for the brain.

When the blood-sugar sensory receptor cells are destroyed in the hypothalamus, the same obesity syndrome in the rats with VMH lesions and victims of Prader-Willis syndrome occurs. This backs up the theory that the sugar receptors in the VMH receive information about blood sugar levels. The VMH observations, therefore, also fit in with the glucostatic theory of hunger.

Researchers have shown that when people feel hungry, their blood-sugar level is low, and when they are not hungry, their blood-sugar level is high. In normal people, the pancreas gland releases insulin, a hormone that enables the tissues of the body to use blood sugar. Without insulin, blood sugar is not taken into the cells but remains in the blood, building up to very high levels. In diabetes, the pancreas falls down on the job of producing enough usable insulin, resulting in high blood-sugar levels and tissue starvation. (A sudden drop in weight is often the first symptom of diabetes.) If you were not hungry and you were given a dose of insulin, thus lowering your blood-sugar levels, you would become hungry just as if you had gone for some time without eating. Thus, a drop in blood-sugar level is a stimulant to start eating. Conversely, a high blood-sugar level would make you want to stop eating. The latter effect is the basis for a weight-reducing diet that provides candy thirty minutes before meals. The idea is that the candy will reduce your appetite at mealtime.

Diabetics, whose problem is chronic high blood-sugar levels, still become hungry, so there must be other factors besides blood sugar involved.

Since energy is stored as fat, logically, the brain should be told how much reserve energy it has in storage. Dr. Mayer came up with the lipostatic theory as a complement to his glucostatic theory. The specific substances by which the body knows how much fat it has in the bank, he hypothesized, are free fatty acids. When the circulating levels of free fatty acids are high, as would be the result of the breaking down of stored fat, we increase our food consumption. When they are low, indicating that fat is being stored rather than utilized, we eat less. Your body, so the theory goes, knows about the level of free fatty acids because your brain's hypothalamus has sensory receptor cells that detect fatty acids just as it has sensory receptor cells that detect sugar. Working in concert with the sugar detectors, these nerve cells may activate the hunger system in your brain to make you start eating.

Both the glucostatic and the lipostatic theories are based on the idea that your body works to maintain a constant value in temperature, blood sugar, salt, and oxygen—known as *homeostasis*. Sensors in your body detect any deviations and make your body take action to recover the normal set-point. Such systems operate by means of negative feedback from the sensors in your body to a central control in your brain.

The fat you store in your body is believed to help your brain decide your personal set-point—the weight at which you stabilize. Some researchers say that if you vary too much from this set-point, gaining or losing too much weight, your brain will direct your body to defend against the radical change and restore the set-point. It will accomplish this by holding back or releasing stored fat and by making you want to eat or not want to eat.

The concept of set-point is useful in understanding how your brain, your autonomic nervous system (which regulates automatic activities such as your breathing and heart action), neurotransmitters (which send messages between your brain cells), and hormones (which transmit messages between glands) act in unison to regulate these and other functions. There are now believed to be two signal systems for hunger and satiety:

1. Signals are sent out when food passes through your gastrointestinal tract.

2. Signals are sent from your brain that integrate the information from your gut signals and send out further instructions.[8]

THE MEAL MESSENGERS—HORMONES AND NEUROTRANSMITTERS

The link between your brain's hypothalamus and your gastrointestinal tract is the object of a tremendous amount of research today. Some investigators refer to it as "the brain in the gut." They want to know why chemical "signals" commonly found in our intestines are also in our brains.

Gastrin, a hormone secreted by the lower part of your stomach when it is full of food, is just such a chemical signal. Gastrin then travels into your blood stream and acts on the upper part of your stomach to stimulate the production of gastric acid. Gastrin is also one of the gut proteins recently found in the brain. To determine if gastrin in the hypothalamus might influence digestion, researchers at the University of Western Ontario injected it into the hypothalamus of rats and then measured stomach acid secretion. Gastrin consistently caused stomach acid secretion to double or triple within fifteen minutes. In contrast, injection of other chemical signals common to the gut and brain did not increase stomach acid. The researchers believe that brain gastrin influences the gut by acting as a neurotransmitter on the vagus nerve, which connects the brain and stomach. When the investigators severed the vagus nerve in rats, brain gastrin did not increase stomach acid.[9]

CCK, another chemical signal, is a local hormone released from your gut during the early stages of your digestion of fats and proteins. It acts as a powerful suppressant of normal eating. CCK also appears to act on the vagus nerve and is found in many place in the brain. administration of CCK to human volunteers reduced meal duration and intake.[10] CCK is sold in health food stores as an appetite suppressant, but many researchers believe that its ability to cause nausea is its real effectiveness in dulling hunger.

Norepinephrine is a neurotransmitter that decreases food intake in animals when injected into the hypothalamus. Norepinephrine levels increase in this same brain region when food is injected into the duodenum (the beginning of the small intestine). These results are consistent with the belief that satiety is affected by neurotransmitters in the brain that become activated when food enters the small intestine.[11] Another bit of evidence that norepinephrine may affect satiety is related to the fact that amphetamines, very similar in structure to norepinephrine, were once highly successful "diet pills" until their side-effects and abuse caused the FDA to forbid their use.

The neurotransmitter *serotonin,* which regulates mood, may also be involved in the production of satiety, several studies have shown. It has been reported that overweight people have a lower level of serotonin in their brains, which may be a reason why they have trouble stopping eating. Studies of food intake with fenfluramine, a widely used prescription diet pill with a structure similar to serotonin, have demonstrated that fenfluramine can suppress food intake.[12]

Vasoactive intestinal peptide (VIP) is present in both your brain and your gut. Its duties include lowering your blood pressure by causing dilation of blood vessels, suppressing secretion of your stomach acid, and stimulating secretions in your small intestine and colon. VIP is believed to be a neurotransmitter that plays a role in arousal, a state of mind necessary when hunting food.

Calcitonin is a calcium-lowering hormone released from your thyroid and by your gut after a meal. It has been shown to have a potent hunger-dampening effect.

Corticotrophin-releasing factor (CRF) causes the release of "stress" hormones from your adrenal gland that increase your heart rate and blood pressure and cause the release of a number of hormones from your pituitary gland. Stress, as we all know from experience, can result in increased eating or loss of appetite. When CRF was injected into the brains of rats, it resulted in increased grooming activity, a known response to stress. It also suppresses drinking and feeding behavior under a variety of conditions. Patients with anorexia nervosa have been found to have an overactive hypothalamus, pituitary gland, and adrenal gland, suggesting the basic defect may be an increase in CRF. Similarly, depressed patients, who often have a poor appetite, also have an overproduction of pituitary and adrenal gland hormones, suggesting the possibility of CRF malfunction. Thus it would appear that stress can either produce overeating through activation of the neurotransmitters in the brain or decreased eating through an increase in CRF.[13]

IS IT ALL IN THE LIVER?

Can your liver really be the source of your hunger? Your liver is a chemical processing plant that can switch products very quickly and dramatically when you eat or fast.[14] In contrast, the supply of fuels to your brain do not seem to change that quickly. The liver is also well situated in your body to evaluate your food intake and the supply of fuels in your body.

Evidence that the liver is involved in hunger and satiety stems largely from studies showing that nutrients suppress food intake in animals more effectively when infused directly into the vein leading to the liver than when injected into veins leading elsewhere in the body. Furthermore, intravenous infusions of fructose, a sugar that is not readily utilized by the brain but is used by the liver, reduce food intake in rats, while infusions of beta hydroxybutyrate, which can be utilized by the brain and not by the liver, have little or no effect on food intake.[15]

GASTROINTESTINAL DISTENSION

There are still more signals that affect your hunger. One of the earliest satiety signals proposed and still an active candidate is the filling of the stomach and intestines with non-nutritive bulk—no-calorie material that is given either before or with a meal. This is the theory behind the use of a bubble that is inserted into the stomach and inflated to cause a sensation of fullness. One of the latest models is called the Garren-Edwards Gastric Bubble, developed by a husband-and-wife team of stomach specialists, Lloyd and Mary Garren of Santa Ana, California. The bubble remains in the stomach up to four months, during which three to four pounds per week are lost.

A MATTER OF TIMING

Preloads are substances, such as candy, that are given before meals to induce satiety.[16] Timing is important. Investigators have shown that hunger is best suppressed when the interval between the "preload" and the meal was five to thirty minutes. When the load was given simultaneously with a test meal, the amount eaten was more than when the preloads were given before the meal. This also explains why you are advised when dieting to eat slowly and put down your fork between bites. Time is needed for the chemical signals mentioned in this chapter to fully activate in your brain.[17]

Incidently, during preload tests, it was discovered that soup was more effective in suppressing later food intake than crackers, cheese, and juice.[18]

Another interesting observation about timing concerns the period between your meals. Charles Pollak, M.D., of Cornell University Medical School's Chronobiology Center in Westchester observed patients who lived in a suite of rooms for two weeks without any time cues—no clocks, windows, or routine. Some of the people had a thirty- to forty-hour day-night cycle instead of the usual twenty-four- to twenty-five-hour one. They would stay awake twenty hours and sleep twenty hours. They also separated their meals roughly in proportion to the day, so that the hours between meals were doubled. "They had no absolute knowledge of time. All they knew was they were hungry for lunch," Dr. Pollak says. "As far as we can tell, they are perfectly normal people."[19]

It may be that there are many of us whose meal timing is off from our true biological clocks. We eat because the clock tells us to eat, not because our brains do.

HYPOTHALAMIC THEORY OF THIRST

We have described a great deal of the research that is going on to determine why we eat and stop eating. Perhaps even more important is why we drink and why we stop drinking. Your tissues require an external supply of water. Your brain must detect this need and direct you to obtain it. Your body constantly loses water through breathing, sweating, and the elimination of wastes. This water must be replaced. From eating, your body can conserve supplies of food as fat, but your body's reserves of water are scant. You could go without food for several months, but you would die if deprived of water for even a few days.

It is also possible for your tissues to be overloaded with water. Your brain must be able to direct elimination of an excess, or you would sicken and eventually die if the situation were not corrected.

There are cells in the same region of your brain associated with eating, the hypothalamus, that are called *osmoreceptors*. When these water sensors are stimulated electrically, drinking occurs. If these cells are destroyed, drinking behavior is disturbed.

A further indication that the hypothalamus is the central link for water regulation is its role in the release of *antidiuretic hormone* (ADH or vasopressin). When this hormone is released by your brain, water is retained by your kidneys. The hypothalamus releases ADH both when the water receptors in the brain indicate a fluid loss within the cells and when the pressure sensors, or *baroreceptors,* in the blood vessels indicate a fluid loss between the cells.[20]

Let's say you are working in the garden in hot weather. You sweat and lose a lot of water stored around your cells. The water in your blood pours out to replenish what you have lost. Your kidneys detect this decrease in water and secrete a chemical in your blood that is carried to your brain telling you that you are thirsty, so that you will drink and resupply your body's water. As with eating behavior, your hypothalamus contains two discrete drinking areas: a "start-drinking" area and a "stop-drinking" one. Electrical or chemical stimulation of the appropriate center will result in starting or stopping drinking. Surgical removal or disconnection of the appropriate area will produce an animal that will not drink or one that drinks to excess.

Thirst and hunger are not independent of each other.[21] When eating begins, a great variety of signals are produced, many of which have been implicated in making you drink. These signals include your body's release of histamine, which simulates stomach juices, and insulin, which processes starches and sugars.

If you are deprived of food, you will consume less water. Likewise, if you are thirsty, you will eat less food. Both may be related to the ratio of the weight of food to the weight of water that you tend to keep in your stomach.

Thirst and hunger also interact because many foods contain at least some water, and many liquids contain at least some nutrients, Thus, eating can help satisfy thirst and drinking can help satisfy hunger. For example, you are unlikely to feel hungry after drinking a large chocolate milk shake, and are unlikely to feel thirsty after eating large amounts of lettuce (lettuce is 96 percent water).[22] This also explains why soup was so effective in diminishing appetite in the preload studies described on page 211.

THE DRY-MOUTH THEORY

The "dry-mouth" theory proposes that you want to drink merely because your mouth is dry.[23] This seems to be borne out in patients awaiting surgery. They are not permitted to drink, but if they rinse their mouth out with water, their thirst is often quenched. This is called "sham drinking."

Against this premise is the fact sham drinking does not satisfy thirst.

The general consensus now is that the dry mouth is a signal of thirst but not a cause, in the same sense that stomach contractions are a signal of hunger.[24]

Angiotensin, a powerful elevator of blood pressure, is believed to be another signal for drinking. It is produced by the action of renin, a kidney enzyme. All of the components of the renin-angiotensin system have been found in the brain, and there are indications this system is part of the brain's mechanism for regulating blood pressure. Water deprivation lowers blood pressure and increases salt concentration in the blood. These change are detected by the kidney, which then secretes renin. When renin comes into contact with the blood, angiotensin is produced. Consequently, angiotensin levels are high in your blood when you are deprived of water. Experiments have been shown that when angiotensin is injected into a vein or applied directly to the brain, thirst increases. Angiotensin may be the messenger between your body and brain when your body water falls too low and you should start drinking to replenish it.[25]

Scientists are learning more and more about how hunger, thirst, and satiety centers in the brain work. Sometimes the investigations are dramatic.

Take the case of Peter, a thirty-seven-year-old man who went to two physicians because he was concerned about his habit of raiding the refrigerator three to five times every night. When Peter and his wife went on vacation, they would place food and drink beside the bed every night. Studies at a sleep lab over six nights showed that the nocturnal food forays coincided closely with periods of rapid-eye-movement (REM) sleep.[26]

REM sleep occurs periodically during the night and is accompanied by great electrical activity in the brain. The authors linked Peter's behavior to that of babies. Research has shown that the demand for food in babies is also associated with REM activity. Infants awake periodically to be fed during the night, but adults usually suppress this rhythmic, night-time food pattern.

An even more dramatic example of the brain's control over eating and satiety concerned a thirty-two-year-old woman, Lucy, who was six-feet tall and weighed 405 pounds. Her severe obesity posed a grave risk to her health. No conventional method helped her lose weight. Electrodes were then inserted into her brain through a hole drilled in the top of her skull. (Because the brain has no pain receptors, Lucy was conscious throughout surgery and only a local anesthetic was needed.) A battery-powered stimulator was implanted under the skin in her chest and connected to the electrodes by wires under the skin. Similar techniques to control pain and epilepsy have been used.

During the next four months at home, Lucy used the brain stimulator almost continuously. The doctors readjusted the stimulator periodically to achieve comfortable but effective levels. During this time, Lucy lost thirty-two pounds.

Then she alternated periods with the stimulator on and off. During the time it was on at high level, her caloric intake was markedly lower than when the device was turned off. There were, however, dramatic changes in brain metabolism. Sugar with a radioactive tracer was injected into her arm and a device called a PET scan was used to reveal how her brain was using the sugar. On days when the stimulator was on, overall brain metabolism was about 35 percent higher than when it was off. There were also psychologic side effects during the period of high stimulation. Lucy experienced increases in anxiety, depression, and fatigue as well as clear decreases in friendliness and vigor.[27]

The researchers said the study showed that stimulation of the VMH can be effective in reducing caloric intake. Compared to other surgical procedures, they said, it is relatively safe. However, they noted that the use of the stimulator seems to produce the same emotional problems as other types of weight-loss regimens.

As it is with many bodily processes, we can learn much from patients like Peter and Lucy and from others who have abnormal or exaggerated eating patterns. The following are descriptions of common eating disorders and new findings and theories about what happens with the brain's appetite and satiety controls go haywire.

SELF-STARVATION OR BINGING

Anorexia nervosa is a disorder of unknown cause that occurs most often in young women who starve themselves because of a morbid fear of gaining weight. They are depressed and tend to exercise excessively. Their preoccupation with food usually prompts strange food-related rituals: crumbling food, cutting it into tiny pieces, and not eating with the rest of the family. The anorexic sometimes becomes a gourmet cook, preparing elaborate meals for others while eating low-calorie food herself. The anorexic may have trouble sleeping. As her obsession increasingly controls her life, she may withdraw from friends.

Many of the anorexic's peculiar behaviors and bodily changes are typical of any starvation victim. Thus, some functions are often restored when sufficient weight is regained. Meanwhile, the starving body tries to protect its two main organs, the brain and heart, by slowing down or stopping less vital bodily processes. Thus, menstruation ceases, often before weight loss becomes noticeable; blood pressure and respiratory rate slow; and thyroid function diminishes.[28]

Bulimia is an eating disorder whose victims typically gorge huge amounts of high-calorie food, then purge by vomiting or the use of laxatives and diuretics, excessive exercise, and fasting. National estimates show that as many as six million Americans may be bulimic or bulimarexic, a combination of bulimic and anoretic, with as many as one out of five college-aged women experiencing the disorders.[29]

In addition to mood swings and episodes of weakness, dizziness, and headaches, bulimics suffer potassium deficiencies, stress on their hearts, loss of tooth enamel, irregular heartbeat, constipation, ruptured stomach linings and digestive problems.

While anorexics can starve themselves to death, bulimics may have a mild or marked weight loss. About 90 percent of the anorexic and bulimic population is female.[30]

When anorexia is combined with bulimia, the degeneration can be rapid. Karen Carpenter, the singer, was a bulimarexic. She died of syrup of ipecac abuse. Ipecac is used to induce vomiting. Building up over time, ipecac irreversibly damaged her heart muscle, which eventually lead to her death.

In the past, anorexia and bulimia were thought to be environmentally induced—a problem of emotional attachments and detachments. Researchers, however, are finding more and more abnormalities in the brain's chemical messenger system.

Researchers such as Walter Kaye, M.D., and his group at the University of Pittsburgh School of Medicine have measured the levels of corticotropin-releasing factor (CRF) in the spinal fluid of patients both during anorexia and after weight gain and recovery. A significant correlation was found between the levels of CRF, which turns on the adrenal glands' release of a hormone involved in sugar metabolism, and stress and depression in these patients. CRF levels have also been found to be high in patients suffering from classical depression.[31]

Sarah Leibowitz, Ph.D., an associate professor of neuropharmacology at the Rockefeller University in New York City, and her colleagues believe that anorexics also have a problem with the brain transmitter norepinephrine.

We believe young women with anorexia have a loss, or at least a decrease, of norepinephrine activity in the middle of the hypothalamus, where hunger is stimulated. We think that young women with anorexia may be so desperate to control their appetites, and refuse to consistently to "hear" hunger signals, that they actually end up changing their norepinephrine levels and thus the number of cell receptors on the hypothalamus. Deprived of food, their bodies may put out so much norepinephrine that the middle of the hypothalamus will hastily reduce the number of its receptors to make the "I'm hungry" message less strident. The brain then may make more norepinephrine, the hypothalamus follows by getting rid of more receptors and eventually so much norepinephrine may be expended that the supply runs out. Or, perhaps the hypothalamus reduces its receptors so efficiently that it can no longer respond to the call for food. Whatever happens, the feeling of hunger practically vanishes.[32]

Dr. Leibowitz maintains that we can all control our brains to some extent. Anorexics apparently teach theirs to shut off hunger signals.

The Rockefeller researcher says binge eating occurs in up to 50 percent of anorexic patients. These episodes are associated with greatly increased subjective hunger and frequently are accompanied by breathlessness, sweating, heart palpatations, racing pulse, and inflated metabolic rate. All of these symptoms suggest a general increase in nervous system activity. During the binge, a large amount of food is rapidly consumed in a short time, with a specific preference for high-caloric, sweet-tasting foods. The binge is ended by stomach pain and frequently self-induced vomiting, and results in a depressed mood, feelings of guilt and remorse, and a continuation of the severely restrictive diets typical of the self-starver.

From this brief description of alternate binges and fasts, Dr. Leibowitz says, one becomes acutely aware that anorexia nervosa is not so much a disorder of appetite loss as it is one of increased desire to eat—perhaps specific foods—associated with a profound self-denial of that desire and then periodic breakdowns of the inhibition.

Dr. Leibowitz says that a variety of studies have indicated that anorexia and bulimia are associated with abnormal regulation of sugar and starch ingestion. Anorexics specifically avoid carbohydrate-rich foods, whereas bulimics focus their binging on high-carbohydrate foods. Drugs known to potentiate food intake and hunger in people have also been found to increase the preference for sugars and starches.

There is evidence that glucose tolerance is impaired in anorexics, Dr. Leibowitz says. Anorexics can't utilize insulin effectively, even after they regain weight.

In anorexia, disturbed hormonal rhythms have also been detected. Furthermore, in anorexics, the normal 24-hour pattern of eating behavior appears to be altered, with binging episodes generally occurring at night. Although the basis for these findings is unknown, it is of interest that in rats, norepinephrine and adrenal hormone levels follow a circadian rhythm and are at their peak at a time when eating behavior is normally at a maximum. For nocturnal animals such as the rat, this occurs at the beginning of the dark cycle, when carbohydrates rather than proteins are preferred.

"The relationship of these hormonal changes to the disturbed patterns of eating behavior in anorectics has not been determined," Dr. Leibowitz points out. "However, in normal human subjects, there is some evidence that the adrenal hormone, cortisol, is released at certain times during the 24 hour cycle, and must remain at normal levels for the nerve cells in the brain's hypothalamus to function properly and thus produce normal eating behavior."[33]

As described earlier, anorexia and bulimia are syndromes that involve self-starvation as a predominant feature. In contrast to true anorexics, who systematically restrict their food intake to the point of life-threatening emaciation, bulimics exhibit frequent episodes of binging—particularly carbohydrate-rich foods—which may alternate with periods of self-starvation. Numerous studies, particularly in animals, show that food deprivation—which is known to release the adrenal hormone *corticosterone* and to cause a preference for carbohydrates and fats—has been shown to enhance the production of norepinephrine in the middle of the hypothalamus. The desire for sweets and fats after dieting may explain why most weight-loss regimens are failures. Our brains send out the chemical signals that overwhelm us with a desire for sweets or a cheeseburger after we've had low-caloric foods for awhile.

We asked Dr. Leibowitz if there were anything that surprised her during her more than fifteen years of research with neurotransmitters and eating behavior.

> I marvel at how potent a very small amount of these chemicals is. We can modify a whole daily pattern of feeding with a single injection. I marvel at how easy it is to disturb the neurotransmitters.
> We are not sure why some people become anorectic and bulimic. Stress may initiate these problems but it is not the cause.[34]

Dr. Leibowitz points out that, ironically, it is very difficult to change human eating patterns.

Eating habits—a small breakfast, lunch at noon, dinner at six—are very stable.[35]

And that brings us to the most common eating disorder of all, overeating. The National Institutes of Health's definition is that "obesity is an excess of body fat frequently resulting in a significant impairment of health."[36] The NIH experts agree that an increase in body weight of 20 percent or more above desirable body weight constitutes an established health hazard.

At any one time, ten million Americans are on a diet. They spend millions of dollars for books, devices, and diet foods. Most diets work for awhile and then the regimen becomes abandoned and the weight is regained. Instead of sensing the natural hunger and satiety cues provided by their bodies, dieters follow prescribed selections of food, such as an all-fruit diet, an all-grain diet, or a rigid combination of foods, and then they stop one diet and later try another. In fact, some researchers consider this yo-yo dieting an eating disorder.

Can you really control your eating? Should you fight your set-point? New research confirms what many obese people have been saying all along: they can just *look* at food and become fatter. According to Yale psychologist Judith Rodin, Ph.D., "Simply looking at or smelling food can trigger endocrine responses like those produced when the food is actually in the gastrointestinal tract."[37]

Many researchers believe that at least some obese people are more likely to eat in response to external stimuli such as television commercials or the mere sight of food. They are highly responsive to external cues.

In one set of experiments, Dr. Rodin and her colleagues divided formerly overweight subjects into two groups according to their degree of responsiveness to internal and external cues. The subjects came to the laboratory at noon, after not having eaten since the previous evening. A juicy steak was cooked in front of them, and they were told they could eat it. Blood samples that were taken while they watched the steak cooking showed that the externally responsive subjects, regardless of weight, produced significantly greater levels of insulin.

In subsequent experiments, Dr. Rodin found that the magnitude of insulin release was correlated with the palatability of the food. And the more externally responsive the subject, the more the insulin responded to the idea of the tastiness of the food.[38]

If external responders oversecrete insulin in the presence of compelling food cues, Dr. Rodin says, they are often likely to want more calories in order to balance their hormonal output. And what they do eat is more likely to be stored as fat.

Externally responsive people are, in Dr. Rodin's words, "literally turned on" by food. To make matters worse, their metabolic responsiveness is even greater when they are looking at food they feel they must not eat.

Dr. Rodin points out that some physiologists believe that the body's responses when anticipating a food are, in part, reflexive and innate. However, recent research suggests that you can learn to associate the palatability and satiating power of food with the taste, texture, smell, and energy value of the food. After repeated pairings, the body responds before the food is actually digested—in effect, it anticipates the new level of energy. It is a phenomenon similar to Pavlov's dog, which salivated when a bell rang because it had learned to associate the bell with food.

Your appetite and eating are complicated not only by neurotransmitters sending messages between your brain and intestines but also by psychological, physical, and environmental circumstances. There has been a great deal of new research into human appetite and eating behavior, but there is still much to be learned. In the meantime, if you want to help control your appetite, try the following:

Eat slowly. Most diet programs advocate eating more slowly and putting your utensils down between bites. There is scientific evidence to back this up: it takes about twenty minutes for the signals from your stomach to reach the satiety center in your brain.

Use your head. Try to become more sensitive to the feelings of satiety. Don't keep eating just because your mother always told you clean your plate or because you are watching television or talking.

Go for the fiber. Vegetables, fruits, and bran provide a feeling of fullness because of their fiber content. You should not only include them in your meals but also try preloading—eat a baked potato or a few bran crackers about half an hour before your meal, and you probably will eat less when you sit down to dinner.

Don't eat by the clock. Eat when you are hungry. This is often difficult to do when you are in a family or social setting, but you can manage when you are on your own.

Eat lettuce. Lettuce is composed of a lot of water. It helps control hunger, has few calories, and contains plenty of vitamin C.

Stimulate your mind. If you are very interested in a subject and are concentrating on it, you will not be overly concerned with food.

Relax and raise your serotonin levels. You tend to eat less when you are relaxed, probably because the serotonin level in your brain is high enough to allow you to feel satiated.

If you tend to binge or starve, get professional help. Eating disorders may have a basis in hormonal and neurotransmitter imbalance. Help is available. For more information, write to:

AMERICAN ANOREXIA/BULIMIA ASSOCIATION, 133 Cedar Lane, Teaneck, N.J. 07666

CENTER FOR THE STUDY OF ANOREXIA/BULIMIA, 1 West Ninety-first Street, New York, N.Y. 10024

RENFREW CENTER, 475 Spring Lane, Philadelphia, Pa. 19128

EATING DISORDERS PROGRAM, CARRIER FOUNDATION, Belle Mead, N.J. 08502

ANOREXIA NERVOSA AND RELATED EATING DISORDERS, INC., P.O. Box 5102, Eugene, Oreg. 97405.

◄ 12 ►

Choices—Why You Eat What You Do

---

hat did you have for dinner last night? Meat? Fish? A vegetable?

Did you have dessert? Did you have fruit or a sweet such as cake for dessert?

Look at your pantry shelves. Do you have tacos there or sesame oil or a jar of gefilte fish?

Why do you choose to eat the foods you do? Because you like them? Why do you like them?

Whatever your answers to these questions, they are bound to be incomplete. Your food choices are not simple and not fully understood, even by scientists who have devoted their careers to studying diet selection. Your food choices involve your genetic predisposition, your brain's neurotransmitters, the foods that were chosen for you as a child, your education, your experiences, your desires, your health needs, and where and with whom you eat.

Let's start with the biological reasons for your selections.

TASTE AND SMELL

The two senses most involved in your eating and drinking—your chemical perceiving apparatus—are taste and smell.

The molecules you "taste" are suspended in liquid, generally water or saliva. Taste receptors are located primarily on your tongue in specialized structures called taste buds. Although you can identify a great number of dissolved substances as each having a unique taste, these can all be expressed as various combinations of four basic tastes: sweet, sour, salty, and bitter.

Taste exerts some control over what you eat because you either like the taste of something or you don't.

You were born with a "sweet tooth." Scientists have established a few common and, they believe, innate tendencies in infant taste by watching how enthusiastically babies suck on bottles filled with different solutions. In one study, Diana Rosenstein and Harriet Oster of the University of Pennsylvania videotaped two-hour-old infants as they were fed solutions containing sugar, quinine, salt, or citric acid.[1]

Confirming previous findings, the newborns looked content after enthusiastically consuming the sweet liquid and scrunched up their faces in displeasure when they tasted the bitter quinine. Salty and sour tastes triggered less intense reactions.

Researchers, therefore, believe that when you're born, sweet is good and bitter is bad. Your body is designed that way. The reasons lie in evolution. Those of our ancestors who survived did so because they discovered that the parts of plants containing sugars tended to be laden with energy, while those tasting bitter were often poisonous.

Why are newborns basically indifferent to the taste of salt? In recent years, it was theorized that babies developed salt cravings because their baby foods were salted to please their parents' tastes. Gary K. Beauchamp of the Monell Chemical Senses Center, a research institute in Philadelphia, however, says that at around four months, infants naturally develop a preference for moderate levels of salt, apparently a result of delayed maturation of their nervous systems. Salt is also thought to be an innate taste preference because it is needed for the brain and body to function properly.

The chemistry of bitter and sweet is complex, perhaps because substances that evoke bitter or sweet taste sensations are so many and so varied.

Your personal taste was inherited. This has been proven many times in experiments with *phenylthiocarbamide* (PTC). Seven out of every ten people, it has been determined, find that PTC tastes bitter while the rest find it has no taste at all. The ability to taste PTC's bitterness is a hereditary trait.

This hereditary difference in taste can also be apparent with other substances such as saccharin. Some people find the aftertaste of the artificial sweetener so bitter that they avoid it.

Then there are those with fructose intolerance, the inability to digest fruit sugars. If they do eat fruit, they become pale and nauseous and they vomit, develop diarrhea, and eventually may lose consciousness. Therefore, they certainly do not have a taste for fruit.

Many food preferences appear to be inherited as an adaption over the eons to the environment. Some racial groups have difficulty digesting milk, for instance, because of lactose intolerance. The ancestors of these people who do not have the enzyme to process milk came from hot climates where milk would have spoiled and thus been dangerous to drink. On the other hand, these same ancestors would perspire a lot in the heat and needed salt to retain fluid. Their descendants may have a "salt hunger" coupled with a highly efficient mechanism for using minute amounts of the nutrient. This combination served the tropical ancestors well but now produces high blood pressure in the descendants who live in more temperate climates.

Another large component of taste is the activation of pressure receptors in the mouth—the texture of food is an important determinant of its palatability. Foods that are too hot or spicy activate pain receptors.

Just as food and drugs can interact, many chemicals can affect the way your brain registers a taste message. For example, exposure to *sodium lauryl sulfate,* a detergent in toothpaste, makes the acid in orange juice taste bitter and sour. Artichokes can magically make water taste sweet. If you ate the berries from the West African tropical bush synsepalum dulcificum, everything you ate afterward, including lemons, would taste sugary.

Your sense of taste can also produce an interesting brain phenomenon: adaptation. If you eat mouthful after mouthful of a single food, eventually you will be unable to taste it. This is because the receptors in your brain become less responsive after long exposure to a single stimulus. The corollary is that your nervous system responds best to change. Wine tasters and coffee tasters have known this for centuries—that's why they rinse their mouths with water or eat a cracker between tastes, the purpose being to remove any remainder of the previous sip of liquid as well as to maintain their tongue and brain taste receptors in their most sensitive, nonadapted state.

Traditionally, our sense of smell has been considered of minor importance in contrast to that of other animals whose ability to smell is critical to survival. While it is true that we could survive without olfaction, there is increasing evidence that our ability to smell is critical not only to our choice of a diet but also to our enjoyment of life.

How does our sense of smell work? The truth of the matter is that scientists still do not know. They know how we see and hear, but they are mystified about how tiny molecules inhaled from the air can be processed and identified by our brains and how our brains can file away those identifications indefinitely in memory. Investigators are still puzzled about how odorants can trigger drives for sex, aggression, and hunger.

They do know that your nose's most important job is to give you information about your environment. In animals such as the dog, the skeleton of the snout projects well beyond the eyes. In primates such as humans, the bony skeleton of the nose is still present but very much flattened. The difference between the snouts of other animals and the noses of primates is attributed to the latter's move up from the ground to the trees, where most primates remain.

Because primates lived in the trees and developed a grasping hand as opposed to a clawed forefoot, sniffing became less important than good eyesight. As a result, the long snout with which other mammals explore smells on the ground was no longer necessary. As the snout shrank, the nasal barrier between the eyes decreased, allowing the fields of vision to overlap.

In mammals such as rodents and dogs, which depend on smell for survival, the olfactory brain structures are relatively large and occupy all or a large part of the lower-front surface of the brain. But in monkeys, apes, and humans, there is a marked reduction of all olfactory structures.

That is not to say that our noses are unimportant. One very vital function of the nose is to monitor every bite of food we eat. In its position above our mouths, it checks safety through aroma. Bad odor equals bad food. The nose also encourages us to nourish ourselves by the pleasure we derive from delicious-smelling food.

Our sense of taste is powerful. We can identify quinine, for instance, in as little as one-part-per-billion solution. But taste pales next to our amazing ability to smell. We can detect an unlimited number of odors, some from far away and in dilutions as weak as one part in several billion parts air.

Everything has an odor to some degree, but particles for either taste or smell must be soluble. This is a throwback to our ancestral life in the sea, when smell and taste were one. Sugar has no taste on a dry tongue, just as the scent of baking bread would go unnoticed in a dry nose. In order to be smelled, molecules also have to be volatile. They must leave their source and float around in the air, even if the air is still.

When it comes to food, successful cooks know that aroma is the difference between an adequate and a great meal. The term *aroma* usually describes a sensation that is somewhere between taste and smell, although taste itself is primarily smell.

Smell and its sensory companion, taste, affect the functioning of your digestive system via your brain. Stimulation of these senses can trigger the brain centers that initiate eating, influence the volume and character of saliva flow, increase intestinal motility, modify both the volume of pancreatic flow and its protein content, and influence the selection of nutrients.

Some who are deficient in thyroid hormone also gradually lose their sense of smell and taste. They may not know it at first. They may begin to add so much salt and sugar to food that they may adversely affect their health and, if they prepare meals, that of their family's as well.

No wonder patients with underfunctioning thyroid glands show very little interest in eating and frequently complain of loss of appetite.

"It is a common misconception on the part of the general public," according to Dr. Richard S. Rivlin of Columbia University, "that an underactive thyroid gland or slow metabolism is the cause of obesity. In overweight patients, the thyroid is nearly always normal."[2]

After treatment with thyroid hormone, he said, every patient reported appetite improvement. In most cases, the patients noted themselves that their smell and taste sensations increased.

In the animal kingdom, the selection of food is rather simple. Eating is a function of the fulfillment of a purely physiological need as well as of the availability of food. But with humans, the decision is rather complex. We eat not only to live but also for a variety of other reasons. A shared meal, for instance, can afford excellent social contact—hence the business lunch and the dinner party. Various factors enter into the choice of a meal, including cost and cultural preference, but aroma, sight, and touch are the most basic.

If food were to taste alike and the only distinction was in texture, eating would be boring. As food becomes scarcer and more of it is manufactured and stored over a long period of time rather than bought fresh and cooked at home, there will be an increasing need to preserve natural aromas or add artificial ones. A food must smell fresh. Increased understanding of the connection between human food choices and food odors will be extremely important. It is no coincidence that bakery departments are frequently placed near the door of supermarkets. The smell literally turns on the taste buds and compels you to buy.

Overall, taste and smell are essential though not infallible guides for monitoring the intake of food. There are many other biological and cultural reasons you select the foods you do, and these reasons often overlap. The innate wisdom of the chemical senses can be overridden by many factors in your life.[3]

BRAIN MECHANISMS AND CRAVINGS—FOOD PREFERENCES

It's 10:00 P.M. and you have a craving for a ham sandwich. It's 10:00 A.M. and you are longing for a jelly doughnut and a cup of coffee.

We mentioned binge eating as part of bulimia in chapter 11, but most of us frequently have a compelling urge to eat a particular item. Food cravings can crop up at any time for any number of reasons including pregnancy, menstruation, and stress.

A craving could also be a signal that your body's store of a certain nutrient is running low, especially if it is for a food you normally don't select. This can happen when you are on a stringent diet and you suddenly crave a high-fat food such as a cheeseburger. There is evidence that when you lose a lot of weight, your fat cells shrink and they try to plump up again by signaling your brain to get the cheeseburger.

A late-afternoon craving can be a signal to your body that your blood sugar is low and that it's time to eat again. Hence the British tea and the afternoon American snack habits.

Cravings can also be switched on by emotions. Early associations with sweets and comfort or rewards often stick with us when we grow up.

Salt appetite is one of a group of so-called specific hungers that are known to develop in states of need. The classic case is the report of a three-and-a-half-year-old boy with adrenal insufficiency who ate copious amounts of salt until he was deprived of it in the hospital, whereupon he suddenly died. Salt craving has been reported in persons on extreme low-sodium diets and as a result of a negative sodium balance resulting

from excessive water drinking. Increased salt preferences may also occur
in the early stages of more moderate sodium-restricting diets, although
the attraction to the taste of salt decreases after a few months.[4]

HORMONE CRAVINGS

The hormonal shifts of menstruation and pregnancy are often behind
certain cravings. Studies show that many women eat chocolate right
before and during their periods.

Pregnancy, too, can spark colorful cravings, most commonly explained by the fact that the developing baby depletes its mother of
calories and nutrients, which the mother's body then craves, says Dr.
Schiffman. Take the classic maternal mania for ice cream, milk, and
other dairy products, then consider this: requirements for calcium, one
of the most necessary nutrients for fetal development, go up 50 percent
during pregnancy.

You can also be turned off by foods during pregnancy. This may be
a primitive protective mechanism, since they are often foods high in
proteins and fats. In ancient times, without refrigeration, these types of
food would have spoiled easily.

Somehow the body instinctively detects the potential risk and turns off
more easily to certain substances such as alcohol and caffeine, both of
which are known for their potential fetus-harming effects. Women who
listen to their bodies often avoid drinking either.

But for the most part, these types of food aversions are learned, usually
from feeling nauseated or getting sick after eating something—even if the
food wasn't the cause of the queasiness. In fact, Paul Schulman, Ph.D.,
an associate professor of psychology at State University of New York's
College of Technology at Utica-Rome, found that pregnancy-triggered
aversions usually occur during the first three months, when morning
sickness is most likely to occur.[5]

Sarah Leibowitz, Ph.D., of Rockefeller University, New York City,
says we do have specific appetites for things. We do like salt and carbohydrates. These cravings are controlled through the brain. Reducing
serotonin levels suppresses the appetite for carbohydrates, and we have
found that if we inject a certain brain chemical, neuropeptide Y, into the
brains of animals, they crave carbohydrates.[6]

She and the other researchers at the forefront of the study of brain and eating behavior agree that the interaction is complex. One of the classic examples involves rates who were deficient in the B vitamin thiamine. Initially, it was demonstrated that thiamine-deficient rats could make appropriate dietary choices to alleviate the vitamin deficiency. Given a choice of three foods, one supplemented with B vitamins, rats deficient in vitamin B quickly came to choose the enriched food whereas the nondeficient controls did not. Subsequently, it was shown that thiamine-deficient rats display an inclination to sample new foods at well-spaced intervals. The spacing allowed time for the benefits of the thiamine supplementation to take effect. The animals were able to make the connection between the thiamine-enriched food and the fact that they felt better. They behaved logically and learned to correct their vitamin deficiency by chosing the enriched food.[7]

In the 1920s, Clara Davis, a pediatrician, began conducting a series of studies to see if, among other things, "young children could choose their diets and thrive without adult direction as to just what and how much to eat."[8] What she found was that when offered a variety of nutritious foods, infants and toddlers instinctively selected foods in combinations that were sufficient for growth and maintenance of health and vigor. Dr. Davis planned to take her research one step further by offering children a choice between nutritious foods and sweet but nutrient-lacking items such as cake and candy. But the Great Depression intervened and prevented her from finishing her work.

Despite the fact that Dr. Davis was never able to complete her studies, her initial research fostered the popular belief—even among physicians—that children know instinctively what to eat, no matter what foods are put before them. That is a myth. Mary Story, Ph.D., R.D., of the University of Minnesota School of Public Health, points out that when children are given a choice between nutritious food and sweet-tasting but nutrient-lacking items such as pastry and ice cream, chances are they will opt for the sweets.[9] That is because children are born with an innate preference for sweets, as pointed out earlier in this chapter.

The flavor cravings of some obese people can be due to their association of the taste of food with its pharmacologic effects. Persons who crave sweets are often addicted to what they describe as a "sugar rush." Sugar turns on the sympathetic nervous system and carbohydrates can increase serotonin levels in the brain. The result is diminished pain sensitivity and decreased appetite. The amino acid tyrosine in food has antidepressant effects. Food can even stimulate the endorphins, the pleasure molecules in the brain. Thus, our taste and desire may simply reflect a need to modify our mental state.

Food preferences, however, can be affected by where you are and with whom you are eating. Many of us prefer to eat the same foods our dinner companions select. Indeed, many people would argue that human food habits are dominated by ethnic, racial, cultural, sociopolitical, and economic factors that collectively overwhelm any basic biological dispositions. In certain cases, for example, political hunger strikers will ignore their bodies' needs and starve themselves to death.

Diet has always been influenced by nonnutritional factors, including geography, economic and technological development, and a host of often subtle cultural determinants. Religious taboos, social status, ethnicity, and sex roles have helped shape our dining patterns. For example, the longstanding preference for wheat as against rye, corn, or oat bread throughout most of the western world has its origins in the religious rites of antiquity. Sex-role identification is evident in the American "meat and potatoes man" and the feminine identification with vegetables, salads, and tea.

Bertram M. Gordon, Ph.D., says in *Nutrition Today* that the act of eating is far more than simply a physical ingestion of food; it is filled with ritual significance. Meals have structures deeply routed in the past.[10]

Anthropological studies tell us much about the impact of culture on food-oriented behavior and nutrition. For one thing, a wide range of nutritious foods are eaten by cultures around the world, but each culture eats only a portion of the available foods and most have customs and practices that ban certain nutritious foods. Some outstanding examples include the pig in Moslem and Jewish cultures, the sacred cow in India, and horse meat in France and the United States.

Some food practices represent a wisdom of the sociocultural system evolved over the generations, such as eating combinations of foods like beans and corn, where the missing tryptophan in corn is supplied by the beans. Sometimes, of course, the "wisdom" may not be so wise, as in the case of societies where polished rice is preferred to whole-grain rice as a dietary staple. Other food practices, especially flavoring and spicing, even with initially distasteful substances such as chili pepper, may serve as a cultural marker of safe and familiar food.

Meat dishes were associated with heroism in the Homeric epics of ancient Greece. Accordingly, meat was for an aristocratic warrior class rather than the poorer peasants. Skeletons of aristocrats were found to have been three inches taller than those of the commoners in ancient Greece. The poor usually ate little more than coarse bread.

As Greece evolved toward the classical period of the age of Socrates, Plato, and Aristotle, the "symposium"—the evening meal with lots of food and good talk—became the center of literary and philosophical discourse, and a more refined dining style succeeded that of the rougher Homeric age. Spartan austerity was reflected in the food eaten there; a black broth of pork stock, vinegar, and salt. After sampling this fare, one contemporary visitor remarked that it was no surprise that Spartans were willing to risk their lives in battle. Death was obviously preferable to life on such a regimen.[11]

Dr. Gordon says that, today, our culture is preoccupied with food processing. Already in vogue is the term *engineered foods* in reference to meat made of vegetable protein and other products. In a larger sense, the term describes the entire gamut of processed foods and the current revolt toward simpler "natural" or "health foods" or toward foreign cuisines reflects a rebellion against social engineering in the solutions of political and social problems. Many of the young middle-class rebels who were against the social engineering policies at home and abroad a decade ago have become the older natural-food enthusiasts and gourmet home cooks resisting an omnipresent food engineering, whose proponents dominate the mass media.

"Food practices," says Dr. Gordon, "continue to mirror social and cultural values as they have since the beginnings of our civilization. They embrace a system of meaning and values that transcend the material content of the food and the ways in which it affects our bodies."[12]

Food is connected with many significant events in our lives. It can be an expression of love and friendship and an important feature of holiday and other celebrations. Food and our emotions are strongly connected. When food becomes a means of coping with anger, depression, and feelings of inadequacy and loneliness, the pattern of food abuse becomes addictive and dangerous.

Our cultural attitudes towards fatness and thinness and what is accepted as ideal body weight socially today greatly determines what we select at the supermarket. As Stefani Sheppa, ACSW of the University of Medicine and Dentistry of New Jersey, puts it, "Our society places a great deal of importance on being thin and fit but we are surrounded by gourmet restaurants, bakeries, and ice cream parlors. Cookbooks containing the ultimate in recipes for delicious desserts, breads, and other mouth-watering delicacies top the bestseller lists."

Ms. Sheppa, who is a social worker and directs a woman's support group for eating disorders, concludes, "Surrounded by all this temptation, we are reminded that it is fashionable and attractive we must be pencil slim."

It may be "in to be thin" but it is not easy.

HOW TO MAKE GOOD FOOD CHOICES

Susan Schiffman, Ph.D., of Duke University maintains that one of the main characteristics that distinguishes overweight persons from their leaner counterparts is simply that they want more intense and varied taste, odor, and texture from their food. That is, the obese person has an exaggerated flavor and texture set-point.

"It would appear that each of us, whether thin or overweight, has a set-point for flavor and texture."[13] Dr. Schiffman says. we each must derive a certain level of sensation from food and beverages in order to feel satisfied with what we have eaten. An important question is whether an elevated need for flavor and texture is the result of learning or of genetics. One cause appears to be the experience of dieting itself. Flavor deprivation during dieting, compounded by acclimation to intense and varied levels of flavor during bingeing, can drive the flavor set point higher. This is illustrated by the fact that many dieters yearn for foods like pepperoni pizza after several days of cottage cheese and lettuce. Another reason that overweight people have higher flavor set-points is that they tend to use food to deal with uncomfortable states such as boredom, anger, or frustration. The simple act of eating more accustoms them to greater amounts of flavor during the course of the day.

Dr. Schiffman, who is head of the weight-loss program at Duke University Medical Center, has developed a flavor spray for dieters. In 1987, the Nutri/System company introduced the flavored sprays, each of which contains less than one calorie a shot. The flavor spray is made by conjuring up the chocolate odor, for example, mixing it with water and sorbitol, a low-calorie sweetener, and then putting it in a pocket-sized spray can. "What happens," Dr. Schiffman says, "is that after three sprays, five maybe—some hard core chocoholics may go up to 20 sprays—then you don't want to taste that [flavor] anymore. It's sensory specific satiety."[14]

Even if you emptied the canister, which contains about 150 sprays, the total intake would be only 15 calories. The flavor sprays cost about $2.50 each and come in flavors such as chocolate, peanut butter, and apple cinnamon.

Dr. Schiffman once had a weight problem herself, but now she takes the flavor spray with her to restaurants. "When the chocolate cheesecake comes around, I reach for my spray,"[15] she says.

Taste also has something to do with the weight gained after smokers quit smoking. Some believe that it may be smoking's effect on appetite or metabolic processes. However, Neil Grunberg, Ph.D., and his colleagues at the Uniformed Services University of the Health Sciences, Medical Psychology Department, Bethesda, Maryland, believe it may be because cigarettes kill the desire for sweets. Consumption of these foods increases when smoking ceases, but consumption of salty, bland, and nonsweet, high-calorie foods does not increase.[16]

On the other hand, cigarette smoking and alcohol may make it harder to control cravings for certain foods. Alcohol and the chemicals dissolved in it stimulate receptors throughout the oral cavity and throat and its volatile components stimulate receptors in the nose. Smoke activates temperature receptors as well. People who quit drinking or smoking miss such stimulation and often turn to other sources of flavor, such as fattening foods. Dr. Schiffman recommends cranberry juice as a helpful substitute to replace the stimulation.

Variety can aid or hinder your efforts to control your eating. Overweight people tend to have an excessive need for variety and intensity in texture, taste, and odor. The texture of food—hardness, brittleness, chewiness, viscosity, and fatty—is also important. It should be noted that a preference for oily, greasy, and creamy textures is due not only to how these feel in your mouth but also to the fact that they can deliver high levels of flavor. Since all odorants are fat soluble, fatty foods can deliver more odor sensations than do foods that dissolve only in water. As pointed out before, we have an adaptive mechanism for both our taste and smell that shuts off these senses after a while and lets us concentrate on something else. But this shut-off system seems to be fooled by a several-course meal in which each course is different in smell, taste, and texture. Feeling "full," or satiated, can be postponed by the stimulation of new foods being served.[17]

On the other hand, if you are on a diet and miss certain foods, switch from food to food as you eat, never eating two bites of the same food consecutively, and you can avoid sensory fatigue. But of course you have to control the total amount by limiting portion size.

The reason most diet programs ask you to chew your food longer than you usually do is because chewing releases taste and aroma and gives you more satisfaction from your meal. It also delays your shoving more food in your mouth. It takes fifteen to twenty minutes for the satiety message to reach your brain from your stomach. Eating food warm also seems to help control the amount you eat. And since the taste buds are on the tongue, many dieters have learned that they don't have to swallow what they put in their mouths. You can take something that is fattening, chew it, and spit it out.

Taste buds, of course, present the first line of receptors for food enjoyment. Older people may have a loss of appetite because their senses of taste and smell may decline as they age. Researchers have found that vitamin C supplementation can prevent or delay the decline of the taste buds. Michigan researchers found that one-third of the older women who came in for clinical evaluation had tongue papillae atrophy. They found that those who didn't have the taste-bud loss had significantly higher intakes of vitamin C.[18]

As for the crazy cravings of children, don't make the same mistakes our parents made. Don't force certain foods on your children and don't stop them from eating just one food. Children go on food jags, a normal part of learning to select their own diet.[19]

As this chapter has pointed out, food choices are very complicated. Quite clearly, your brain has the final say over your menu selection.

Millions of dollars are spent each year trying to influence your choices. More than five thousand items a year are introduced to supermarket shelves in hope of luring you into buying them. Not every new product can be a knockout, like light beer or TV dinners. Eighty percent are commercial duds.

One example of misreading the market occurred when Gerber foods tried to market foods for grownups such as beef burgundy and Mediterranean-style vegetables. The company's mistake was to put the food in containers that looked like baby-food jars. Gerber compounded its problem by labeling the product *Singles*. Later research showed that adults generally dislike being pegged as singles who eat alone, even if they do.[20]

◈ 13 ◈

Using Your Brain to
Choose Your Diet

The brain is, after all, an organ, like the kidney, the heart, or the liver, and organs are known to fail because of hereditary factors as well as environmental ones. The answer is probably that to many people the brain is much more than an organ; it is the center of the poetry, the sophistication, the special qualities that make human beings an order of magnitude more complex than the closest related species. To believe that the brain is merely a series of chemical reactions is to denigrate free will, to remove the humans from the responsibility for their actions, to eliminate the relation between sin and guilt. Moreover, the recent findings are just the beginning; many other behavioral characteristics have been analyzed by studies of adopted children and identical twins and by biochemical approaches. Those who dread complexity will try to reduce the new evidence to the old confrontation of extremes: chemistry versus free will, heredity versus environment, fate versus responsibility. In fact, the neurobiological evidence indicates that part of the brain is "hard wired" in advance of birth and part is designed to be plastic and learn from experience.

—DANIEL E. KOSHLAND, JR.

THIS BOOK has been about the "free will" to select a nutritious diet for your brain to protect it and maintain it in the best condition possible based on your "hard-wired" heredity and your malleable life-style. There is increasing evidence that certain foods do have an effect on your brain, and we have tried to explain and analyze some of the many factors involved in those interactions. We have reported current research on such questions as how life-style, age, sex, culture, and economic and social influences affect food choices and what the cause and effect of eating habits may be.

We have described the possible effects that salt, sugar, fat, alcohol, additives, and allergens in the food may have on your brain. We have

235

pointed out the interaction of food and medication on the brain, and we presented some of the research reports concerning food, learning, and memory.

The information is drawn from many scientific fields because research into food and the brain spans many disciplines—from neuroscience to nutritional science to advertising psychology.

What should you eat?

You are a unique human being with your own genetic, social, and medical history, and one of the major purposes of this book is to help you make informed choices for yourself.

SHEDDING LIGHT ON LITE FOODS

As the *Wall Street Journal* pointed out recently, nearly everything that we eat today is being promoted as "healthful" or "natural." Even Spam luncheon meat is being touted as "real pork shoulder." Marketers are responding to the ever-growing cry from consumers for more nutritious food products.

Chicken of the Sea tuna producers, for example, created a new label to make their product seem purer and healthier. The old can said the fish was "packed in water"; the new can says "packed in pure spring water." A Nabisco product shows a cheese wheel on the package and says in big letters, "Now With Real Wisconsin Cheese." Although the product didn't actually change, sales did: they increased.

In a similar move, General Foods changed the name of their Super Sugar Crisp cereal to Super Gold Crisps, although it is the same cereal.[1]

We not only want to be slimmer, we also want to be healthier. *Advertising Age,* the trade journal of those who lure us into buying products, reported recently that the ranks of dieters who just want to lose weight have thinned from 22 percent in 1981 to 19 percent at last count. Those of us who wish to limit salt and cholesterol intake, however, have grown in number. The latest surveys show 13.2 percent of us are on a low-salt regimen, versus 6.5 percent in 1981; 8 percent of us are trying to control cholesterol, compared to 2 percent in 1981.

Responsive to our desires, food producers have quickly brought to market a wide variety of "lite" items, and we've grabbed them off the shelves. When Quaker Oats, for example, wanted to revive Aunt Jemima syrup, the sales of which had been declining for years, the company created a lite version. The *Journal of Consumer Marketing,* a trade publication, reported that Auntie's sales quickly doubled.

What do you believe about a product when you see the word *lite* or *light* on the label? Most of us assume that an item is called lite for one or more of the following reasons:

- Fat ordinarily in the item was reduced or eliminated
- It was baked instead of fried
- Artificial sweeteners or sweeter-tasting compounds were substituted for sugars
- The amounts of sugars and/or starches were reduced
- The amount of salt was reduced or eliminated

Manufacturers, however, are free to use the lite label for other purposes. One salad oil, for example, was labeled lite because it was lighter in color, not in fats or calories.

The word *new* on a package—a tried-and-true marketing ploy—can be used for only six months, but a spokesperson for the FDA points out that there is no time limit on the use of the word *lite* or *light* on labels under current government regulations. There is no legal way to stop a from interpreting the word any way it wishes. A number of processors are promoting new products as lite and lower in calories, fat, and salt when all they have done is to reduce the size of the portions listed for the old products.

How can you determine what is really light?

Food has three major components—protein, carbohydrate, and fat. Carbohydrate—sugars and starches—contributes four calories per gram and so does protein. Fat, however, contains a whopping nine calories per gram.

Fat, because it has correlated with an increased risk of stroke, heart disease, and cancer as well as with those cosmetically undesirable extra pounds, is a prime target for reduction in the diet.

No rules exist, as of this writing, for claims about the saturated fat and cholesterol in a product, although the FDA is in the process of forming such regulations. According to the agency's proposal, the following should be in the package when lower-cholesterol claims are on the label:

- Cholesterol-free = less than 2 milligrams per serving
- Low cholesterol = less than 20 milligrams per serving
- Reduced cholesterol = the new product was reformulated or processed by 75 percent or more compared with the old (for example, cholesterol was reduced from 120 milligrams to 30 milligrams per serving).

If a significant reduction were made, but not as much as 75 percent, the label could still read: "Cholesterol in this pound cake reduced 35 percent—from 70 milligrams to 45 milligrams per serving."

When it comes to meats, the word is often "lean" rather than "lite."

A company can call a meat lean or low-fat if the meat has 25 percent less calories, fat, sodium, cholesterol, or breading. The standard for comparison may be the company's own unreduced product, a government market standard, or a standard industry product.

Chicken has been promoted as containing less fat than red meats. Indeed, a USDA study shows that in a quarter pound of boneless chicken there are 13.6 grams of fat, compared to 20 grams in the same amount of hamburger; and approximately 28 percent of the fat in chicken saturated, compared to 38 percent of the fat in beef. As if that weren't enough, chicken producers are now trying to sell us slim birds. Perdue claims to be producing a chicken 24 percent lower in fat, and Holly Farms touts theirs as having 14 percent less fat.

Sugar is poured into processed foods not only as a sweetener but as a thickener, stabilizer, and coloring agent. Oil and fats are also added to suspend flavorings and spices and to provide a sense of smoothness and fullness.

Advances in food technology have made possible the development of specialized ingredients that have some of the functional properties of sugar, fat, and starch without the high calories. In most cases, they cannot totally replace the ingredient. For example, polydextrose, a bulking agent approved for food use in 1981, has one calorie per gram, is water soluble, and is used to partially replace ordinary sugar and/or fats in baked goods, baking mixes, salad dressings, gelatins, puddings, candies, gum, frozen dairy products, desserts, and mixes. It provides thickness and texture and retains moisture in a variety of foods. In addition, high-fructose corn syrups, which are sweeter tasting than sugar, allow producers to use less sweetener and thus reduce the calories.

Calories may also be reduced by substituting vegetable gums for oils in salad dressings and desserts.

Still another specialized ingredient is powdered cellulose, an almost noncaloric ingredient containing fiber and used as a bulking agent to replace flour in baked goods and to add body to sugar- and fat-free foods.

Then, of course, there are the artificial sweeteners such as saccharin and aspartame. Diet soft drinks represent the largest portion of the diet food and drink market. Should you select artificial sweeteners over sucrose or fructose? Read pages 65–67 and 150–152 and make up your mind.

What about calorie counts on the label? The FDA has the following rules for labels and content:

- Low calorie = no more than 40 calories per serving

- Reduced calorie = fewer calories than in its standard form

A "reduced-calorie" food, therefore, could contain more calories than a food that is naturally low in calories. Consumers should also be wary of the words *sugar-free* on a label. Such items may not contain so-called table sugar but can be high in other forms of sweeteners. Ingredients with the *-ose* ending, as in dextrose or maltose (corn and malt sugars), or *syrup* usually mean there is sugar in an item.

One of the newest entries on the lite market is lower-alcohol-content wines. California wines have about 12 to 14 percent alcohol by volume while German wines have about 8 percent. The lower-alcohol wines, which are expected to contain 10 percent alcohol, will reduce both the calories and the "buzz."

Should you drink any alcohol if you want to protect your brain? After you've read pages 127–128 and 143–148, you can make up your own mind.

Whether you drink to that or not, a final precaution: the word *lite* on a label doesn't give you a license to binge. You can follow a healthy, weight-controlling, and satisfying diet by being enlightened about "lite" claims.

How can you buy wisely? What should you eat?

You may have special needs, depending on your heredity, your health, and your life-style, so the following is merely a general menu from which to choose. The safest bet for most people—both in terms of health and effectiveness—is a well-balanced, varied, low-calorie diet.

A rough way to estimate your personal calorie needs is to estimate your basal metabolism rate (BMR), the rate at which you burn energy at rest. Multiply your current weight by ten. If, for example, you are a woman who weighs 130 pounds, your BMR calorie needs are 1,300. The second calculation you need to make is how many calories you burn a day through your various activities. Because most of us are sedentary, some experts believe you can figure only 30 percent of BMR for activity calories. Thus, unless you are a physically active 130-pound woman, you should add only another 390 calories (.30 × 1,300) to the 1,300 basic level for a total of 1,690 calories to maintain your current weight.

Once you know the daily calorie intake that keeps you at your present weight, you can lose weight by creating a "negative energy balance." Specifically, to lose one pound of fat you need to consume about 3,500 calories less than you use each week. If you cut back 500 calories a day, you'll lose a pound a week.

The main feature of a balanced diet is that although calories are limited you can still choose from a variety of foods—breads and other starches, fruits, vegetables, dairy products, and protein sources such as lean meat and poultry.

For your body and brain, a balanced diet emphasizing more carbohydrates and less protein is recommended.[2]

- Complex carbohydrates such as pasta, bread, cereal, and starch should make up 50 to 60 percent of your calories;

- Protein should constitute about 15 to 20 percent;

- Fats should be 20 to 30 percent of your calories, with two thirds to three quarters polyunsaturated or monounsaturated (see pages 97–98).

There are other wise decisions:

- Eat regionally, because you are more likely to get fresher fruit and vegetables still containing many of their vitamins.

- Cut down on sugar and skip sodas and imitation fruit drinks containing only 10 percent fruit because they are very high in sugar and coloring.

- Eat as many simple, unprocessed foods as possible. Food processing prevents the growth of germs and decay producing organisms, but it uses heat, refrigeration, freezing, radiation, separation methods, gas, alterations in water content, fermentation processes, and packaging, all of which may affect your nutrients. Canned vegetables, for example, contain only 30 to 50 percent of the vitamin C present in the fresh product and may lose up to 20 percent of the vitamin A and thiamine. Part of the loss occurs during blanching before canning. Once a food is canned and stored, there are few changes in its nutritional quality if the product is stored below seventy degrees Fahrenheit. Approximately 25 percent of the vitamin C, however, is lost during one year of storage at seventy to eighty degrees Fahrenheit.

Frozen foods, because they are not treated by heat, have a nutritional quality close to that of the fresh product, except for a loss of 10 to 20 percent of vitamins C, E, and A which occurs during blanching before the freezing process. But factors such as loss of flavor, textural changes, and loss of nutritional value allow only an intermediate shelf life—nine months to one year—for many frozen fruits and vegetables.

For dried foods, the essential amino acid lysine is unavailable for absorption. Browning is a result of the reaction between reducing sugars such as fructose and available amino acid groups found in proteins, as Rockefeller University's Dr. Cerami points out in chapter 10. Since increasing amounts of high-fructose corn syrups are being used as sweeteners in processed foods, this type of browning may prove to be more of a problem.[3]

The following are the basics for a balanced, varied diet: You should have daily, if you wish to have a balanced diet, at least two servings of dairy products such as cottage cheese, yogurt, or milk; two servings of high-protein foods such as lean meat, poultry, fish, eggs, beans, nuts or peanut butter; four servings of fruits and vegetables including citrus fruits or juice and a dark green, leafy vegetable; and four servings of bread or cereal products made with whole-grain or enriched flour, rice, or pasta.

- **Protein** *(two servings per day):* Choose a fish like flounder, instead of chicken, and you'll ingest half the fat and calories. Fresh fish, chicken, turkey, legumes, lean veal, fat-trimmed flank steak, and fat-trimmed leg of lamb are all good choices.

- **Dairy and Oils** *(two servings per day):* Nonfat fortified milk, skim milk, low-fat yogurt; buttermilk (made with skim milk), low-fat cottage cheese; cheeses containing less than percent butterfat; margarine; corn oil; sunflower oil; safflower oil; olive oil; peanut oil; soy oil; ice milk; mayonnaise.

- **Vegetables** *(two to four servings per day):* Select vegetables such as broccoli, cabbage, carrots, tomatoes, cauliflower, watercress, lettuce, corn, and green peppers.

- **Fruits and Fruit Juices** *(two to four servings per day):* Choose fresh, when possible, or canned in their own juices, the following: apples, apricots, bananas, berries, cherries, grapes, oranges, peaches, plums, citrus fruit, fresh fruit juices without added sugar; fruit ice.

- **Carbohydrates** *(four servings per day):* Select whole-wheat, rye, pumpernickel, raisin breads; cornmeal; whole-wheat pasta; brown rice; potatoes (sweet are best), pumpkin, beans, lentils; grits; wheat germ; oatmeal; puffed rice; low-salt crackers.

- **Condiments:** Natural herbs and spices; garlic powder; pepper; lemon juice; fresh onion; tomato; lettuce; cucumber; unsalted, low-fat salad dressing; homemade dressings made with safflower, corn, olive, or cottonseed oil.

- **Treats:** Fresh fruits and vegetables; dried fruits; low-fat yogurt; frozen yogurt; popcorn; homemade oatmeal cookies; raw apples; raisins; ice milk; almonds, walnuts, and peanut butter. Downing one drink of alcohol or devouring a single candy bar is not going to hurt your brain if you do it infrequently and are in reasonably good health.

In the 1980s the American Cancer Society, American Heart Association, and National Institutes of Health all maintained diet can prevent cancer, heart disease, and many other ills. The adage, "you are what you eat" applies not just to heart muscles and bone but to the brain as well. Food fuels your brain and powers its control over your body. Neurotransmitters, those chemical messengers between your nerve cells, are made directly or indirectly from the nutrients you ingest.

What you eat influences the production of the hormones needed by your brain to oversee your body functions, and food provides the vitamins vital to your vitality. Your meals provide substances that your brain requires but cannot make.

This book, we hope, will serve you as a guide to the selection of the nutrients that will help you protect and maintain a healthy brain.

NOTES

INTRODUCTION

1. Robin B. Kanarek, Ph.D., and Nilla Orthen-Gambill, Ph.D., "Complex Interactions Affecting Nutrition-behavior Research," *Nutrition Reviews* 44 (May 1986); 172.
2. Ibid.
3. Ibid.
4. J. Mauron, ed., *Nutrition: Neurotransmitter Function and Behavior* (Toronto: Hans Huber, 1986), 22–23.

CHAPTER 1.
The Brain/Food Connection

1. Timothy J. Maher, "Natural Food Constituents and Food Additives: The Pharmacologic Connection," *Journal of Allergy and Clinical Immunology* 79 (3): 413–21.
2. *Journal of the Florida Medical Association* 47 (1961): 921.
3. Donald S. McLaren, "Vitamin A Deficiency and Toxicity," in *Present Knowledge in Nutrition,* 5th ed. (Washington, D.C.: Nutrition Foundation, 1984), 192–208.
4. M. D. Green, J. Hawkins, and S. T. Omaye, "Effect of Scurvy on Reserpine Induced Hypothermia in the Guinea Pig," *Life Science* 27 (1980):111–16.
5. H. P. Broquist, "Carnitene Biosynthesis and Function," *Fed. Proc.* 41:2840–42.
6. J. M. Feldman and E. M. Lee, "Serotonin Content of Foods: Effects on Urinary Excretion of 5-Hydroxyindoleacetic Acid," *American Journal of Clinical Nutrition* 42 (October 1985):639–43.
7. Phobia meeting, New York, 1986.
8. Raymond Bartus, personal communication with authors, April 15 1985.
9. P. Ferro et al., "A Brain Octadecaneuropeptide Generated by Tryptic Digestion of DBI Functions as a Proconflict Ligand of Benzodiazepine Recognition Sites," *Neuropharmacology* 23(11): 1359–62.

CHAPTER 2.
Amino Acids: Messengers of the Mind

1. John Fernstrom et al. "Diurnal Variations in Plasma Concentrations of Tryptophan, Tyrosine, and Other Neutral Amino Acids: Effects of Dietary Protein Intake," *American Journal of Clinical Nutrition* 32 (September 1979): 1912–22.
2. Andrew Mebane, "L-Glutamine and Mania," *American Journal of Psychiatry* 141 (10 October 1984): 1302–03.
3. "The Case of Too Much Amino Acids," *Tufts University Diet and Nutrition Letter,* 4 (3):7.
4. Carol Ballentine, "The Essential Guide to Amino Acids," *FDA Consumer.* 19(7):23–24.
5. "Beefy Boost For Ailing Immune System," *Medical World News,* 16 February, 1981, 34.
6. E. H. Reynolds, "Folic Acid, S-Adenosyl Methionine and Affective Disorders," *Psychological Medicine,* 13 (4): 705–10.
7. Arthur Winter, M.D., "New Treatment for Multiple Sclerosis," *Neurological and Orthopedic Journal of Medicine and Surgery* 5 (April 1984): 39–43.
8. A. J. Gelenberg et al., "Tyrosine for the Treatment of Depression," *American Journal of Psychiatric Research* 17 (2): 175–80.
9. E. Melamed et al. "Plasma Tyrosine in Normal Humans: Effects of Oral Tyrosine and Protein-Containing Meals," *Journal of Neural Transmission* 47 (1980): 1014–15.
10. Food and Agriculture Organization of the United Nations, Food Policy and Food Science Service, Nutrition Division, *Amino-Acid Content of Foods and Biological Data on Proteins,* (Rome: Food and Agriculture Organization of the United Nations, 1970).
11. L. Vazelli et al., "On the Significance of Tryptophan Content of Foods," *Re-*

search Communications in Psychology, Psychiatry and Behavior 7 (4): 485–88.

12. Ernest Hartmann and C. L. Spinweber, "Sleep Induced by L-Tryptophan: Effect of Dosages Within the Normal Dietary Intake," *Journal of Nervous and Mental Diseases,* 167 (1979): 497–99.

13. Michael Yogman, "Nutrients and Newborn Behavior: Neurotransmitters as Mediators?" *Nutrition Reviews Supplement* 44 (May 1986): 74–75.

14. L. Vazelli, "Tryptophan Content," 485.

15. Elaine D. Nemzer et al., "Amino Acid Supplementation as Therapy for Attention Deficit Disorders," *Journal of the American Academy of Child Psychiatry* 25 (July 1986): 509–13.

16. J. P. Brady, M.D. Cheatle, and W. A. Ball, "A Trial of L-Tryptophan in Chronic Pain Syndrome," *Clinical Journal of Pain* 3 (1): 39–44.

17. "Eating Away Your Pain," *Science News,* 19 February 1983, 125.

18. C. Wayne Callaway, "Nutrition," *Journal of the American Medical Association* 256 (15): 2097–98.

19. John Fernstrom, "Acute and Chronic Effects of Protein and Carbohydrate Ingestion on Brain Tryptophan Levels and Serotonin Synthesis," *Nutrition Reviews Supplement* 44 (May 1986): 25–35.

20. *National Institute of Mental Health Science Reporter,* March 1984, S–3.

21. Paul Teychenne, *Questions and Answers About Parkinson's Disease and its Treatment,* (East Hanover, N. J.: Sandoz Pharmaceutical Co., 1985), 20.

22. J. H. Pincus and K. M. Barry, "Dietary Methods for Reducing Fluctuations in Parkinson's Disease," *Yale Journal of Biological Medicine* 60 (2): 133–37.

23. Ibid.

24. "Change in Diet for Victims of Parkinson's Disease," *Tufts University Diet and Nutrition Letter* 5 (4).

25. Ibid.

26. "Potato Dilemma: To Bake or Fry?" *Science News,* 4 February 1984, 125.

27. Michael Trulson (Paper presented to the 95th Annual Meeting of the American Psychological Association, New York, 31 August 1987).

28. Ibid.

29. National Institute of Child Health and Human Development, "NICHD Guide for Researchers."

CHAPTER 3.
Food: Vitamins, Minerals, and Your Brain

1. "Niacin (Nicotinic Acid) Deficiency" in *Merck Manual,* 14th ed., ed. Robert Berkow (Rahway, N.J.: Merck, 1982), 900–902.

2. Herman Baker, personal communication with authors, 13 February 1987.

3. Frederick C. Goggans, "A Case of Mania Secondary to Vitamin B_{12} Deficiency," *American Journal of Psychiatry* 141 (2): 300–301.

4. Frank Press (Chairman, National Research Council), letter to Dr. James Wyngaarden (Director, National Institutes of Health), 7 October 1985; made public by the National Research Council 7 October 1985, Washington D. C.

5. Food and Nutrition Board, National Research Council of the National Academy of Sciences, "Recommended Daily Dietary Allowances," Revised 1980.

6. Jess Thoene, Herman Baker, et al., "Biotin-Responsive Carboxylase Deficiency Associated with Subnormal Plasma and Urinary Biotin," *New England Journal of Medicine* 304 (April 1981): 817–20; and personal communication with authors, 13 February 1987.

7. Food and Drug Administration, *FDA Drug Bulletin* 9 (November 1979).

8. Baker, personal communication.

9. Ibid.

10. M. Brin, "Dilemma of Marginal Vitamin Deficiency," in *Proceedings of the Ninth International Congress on Nutrition,* 4 (Basel, Switzerland: S. Karger, 1975): 102–15.

11. Ibid.; and M. Brin, "Erythrocytes as a Biopsy Tissue in the Functional Evalua-

tion of Thiamin Status," *Journal of the American Medical Association* 187 (1964): 762.

12. Baker, personal communication.

13. Ibid.

14. H. Baker and O. Frank, *Clinical Vitaminology: Methods and Interpretation* (New York: J Wiley, 1968).

15. Baker, personal communication.

16. Paul Lachance, personal communication with authors, 19 February 1987.

17. C. Michael, R.D. Fisher, and Paul Lachance, "Nutrition Evaluation of Published Weight Reducing Diets," *Journal of The American Dietetic Association,* 85 (April 1985): 450–53.

18. Lachance, personal communication.

19. Ibid.

20. Baker, personal communication.

21. Ibid.

22. William Gottlieb, "Encyclopedia of Vitamins," *Source Book on Food and Nutrition,* (Chicago: Marquis Academic Media, 1982), 86

23. "Hypervitaminosis A," in Berkow, *Merck Manual,* 14: 891.

24. J.. Greenwood et al., "Thiamine, Malnutrition, and Alcohol-related Damage to the Central Nervous System," *Progress in Alcohol Research,* Vol. 1, (Utrecht, The Netherlands: VNU Press, 1985), 287–310.

25. R. Finlay-Jones, "Should Thiamine Be Added to Beer?" *Australian and New Zealand Psychiatric Journal* 20(1) : 3–6.

26. P. F. Nixon et al. "How Does Alcohol Cause Brain Damage?" Report of the Medical Research Advisory Committee to the Australian Associated Brewers, February 1985, 18–24.

27. Vichai Tanphaichitr and Beverly Wood, "Thiamin," in *Present Knowledge in Nutrition,* 5th ed. (Washington, D.C.: Nutrition Foundation, 1984), 273–83.

28. R. J. Harrell, "Mental Response to Added Thiamine," *Journal of Nutrition,* 31 (1946):283.

29. J. Brozek, "Physiological Effects of Thiamine Restriction and Deprivation in Young Men," *American Journal of Clinical Nutrition* 26 (1973): 150.

30. Ibid.

31. M. Brin, "Erythrocyte as a Biopsy Tissue in the Functional Evaluation of Thiamin Status," *Journal of the American Medical Association* 187: 762.

32. M. Brin, "Examples of Behavioral Changes in Marginal Vitamin Deficiency in the Rat and Man" (Paper delivered at *International Nutritional Conference,* Washington D. C., 30 November to 2 December 1977), National Institutes of Health pub. no. 79–1906.

33. Richard Rivlin, "Riboflavin," in *Present Knowledge in Nutrition,* 5th ed., 285–302.

34. B. S. Narasinga Rao, and C. Gopalan, "Niacin," in *Present Knowledge in Nutrition,* 5th ed., 318–31.

35. J. R. Wittenborn, "A Search for Responders to Niacin Supplementation," *Archives of General Psychiatry* 31 (1974): 547.

36. L. M. Henderson, "Vitamin B₆," in *Present Knowledge in Nutrition,* 5th ed., 303–17.

37. H. Schaumburg et al., "Sensory Neuropathy from Pyridoxine Abuse," *New England Journal of Medicine* 34 (suppl. 1):137.

38. Victor Herbert, "Vitamin B₁₂," in *Present Knowledge in Nutrition,* 5th ed., 347–64.

39. Baker, personal communications.

40. V. P. Sydenstricker et al., "Observations on the 'Egg White' Injury in Man and its Cure with a Biotin Concentration," *Journal of the American Medical Association* 118: 1199–1200.

41. Gottlieb, "Encyclopedia of Vitamins," 89.

42. Ibid.

43. Robert E. Olsen, "Pantothenic Acid," in *Present Knowledge in Nutrition,* 5th ed., 377–82.

44. G. Milner, "Ascorbic Acid in Chronic Psychiatric Patients—A Controlled Trial," *British Journal of Psychiatry* 109 (1963): 294–99; and N. Subramanian,

"On the Brain Ascorbic Acid and Its Importance in the Metabolism of Biogenic Amines," *Life Sciences* 20(9): 1479–84.

45. L. C. Tolbert et al., "Effect of Ascorbic Acid on Neurochemical Behavioral and Physiological Systems Mediated by Catecholamines," *Life Sciences* 25(26): 2189–95; G. J. Naylor, "New Approaches to the Treatment of Manic Depressive Illness," *Neuropharmacology* 19: 1233–34; P. Cocchi et al., "Antidepressant Effect of Vitamin C," *Pediatrics* 65(4):862; and Milner, "Ascorbic Acid in Chronic Psychiatric Patients," 294–99.

46. *Merck Manual,* 14: 871.

47. Robert Woods Johnson Medical School, University of Medicine and Dentistry of New Jersey, press release, 10 June 1987.

48. "Lithium: Antidote to Alcoholism?" *Medical World News,* 14 December 1973, 45.

49. Sally Schuette and Hellen Linkswiler, *"Calcium,"* in *Present Knowledge in Nutrition,* 5th ed., 408.

50. Kaymar Arasteh (Paper presented at the 95th Annual Meeting of the American Psychological Association, New York, 31 August 1987).

51. Schuette and Linkswiler, "Calcium," 408.

52. *Merck Manual,* 14:872.

53. F. Xavier Pi-Sunyer and Esther Offenbacher, "Chromium," in *Present Knowledge in Nutrition,* 571–86.

54. E. P. Novikova, "Effect of Different Amounts of Dietary Cobalt on Iodine Content of Rat Thyroid Gland," Federal Proceedings 23 (1963): 1459–60; and R. I. Blokhima, "Trace Elements Metabolism in Animals", ed. C. F. Mills (Edinburgh: 1970), Livingston, 426–32.

55. Eric Underwood, "Cobalt," in *Present Knowledge in Nutrition,* 5th ed., 528.

56. Ronald J. Amen, "Trace Minerals as Nutrients," *Nutrition for Food Executives,* October 1973, 751–56.

57. U. Meri and R. Rahamimoff, "Neuromuscular Transmission: Inhibition by Manganese Ions," *Science,* April 1972, 308–9.

58. Amen, "Trace Minerals," 751–56.

59. Raymond Burk, "Selenium," in *Present Knowledge in Nutrition,* 5th ed., 519–34.

60. Ross M. Welch, U.S. Department of Agriculture Report on Selenium, Washington, D.C., 1986.

61. "Zinc Helps Regulate Chemical Communication Between Brain Cells," *Stanford University Medical Center News Report,* 30 April 1987.

62. Alexander G. Schauss and Derek Bryce-Smith, "Evidence of Zinc Deficiency in Anorexia Nervosa and Bulimarexia," in *Nutrition and Brain Function,* (Basel, Switzerland: S. Karger 1987).

63. Baker, personal communication.

CHAPTER 4. Blood, Brain, and Sugar— How Carbohydrates Affect You

1. "Nutritive Value of Brown, Raw, and Refined Sugar," *Journal of The American Medical Association* 221 (2): 201.

2. Richard K. Bernstein, *Diabetes: The Glucograf Method for Normalizing Blood Sugar* (Los Angeles: Tarcher, 1981), 154.

3. Ibid.

4. Norman Ertel, *Diabetes Care* 8: (May–June 1985): 279–83.

5. Bernstein, *Diabetes,* 154.

6. Ibid.

7. Ruth Winter, *A Consumer's Dictionary of Food Additives* (New York: Crown, 1984), 224.

8. Massachusetts General Hospital, Department of Dietetics, *Energy Modification Diet Reference Manual* (Boston: Little Brown, 1984), 41–61.

9. John Bantle et al., "Postprandial Glucose and Insulin Responses to Meals Containing Different Carbohydrates in Normal and Diabetic Subjects," *New England Journal of Medicine* 309 (1): 7–12.

10. Ibid.

11. "FDA Report Spotlights on Effects of Sugar," *New York Times,* 2 October 1986, C7.

12. Alexander Schauss, "FDA Releases Report of Sucrose and Other Sweeteners: Critics Upset," *International Journal of Biosocial Research,* 8 (2): 109–14.

13. "Hypoglycemia—Fact or Fiction," *Harvard Medical School Health Letter* 5 (1): 1.

14. Ruth Winter, "Do You or Don't You Have Hypoglycemia?" *Glamour,* December 1980, 244–45.

15. National Institutes of Health, "Special Report on Aging," NIH pub. no. 80–2135, August 1980, p. 10.

16. Ibid.

17. Larry Christensen (Paper presented at the 95th Annual Meeting of the American Psychological Association, New York, 31 August 1987).

18. E. Pollitt, R. L. Leibel, and D. Greenfield, *American Journal of Clinical Nutrition* 34 (1981): 1526–33.

19. Anita Lewis (Ph.D. diss., University of Texas at Houston, 1983) *Dissertation Abstracts International* 43 (11).

20. Vicky Rippere, *British Journal of Clinical Psychology* (1983): 314–16.

21. Betty Li and Priscilla J. Schuhmann, *Agriculture Research* (January–February 1980): 15.

22. Angus Craig, "Acute Effects of Meals on Perceptual and Cognitive Efficiency," *Nutrition Reviews Supplement* 44 (May 1986): 163–71.

23. Bonnie Spring et al., "Effects of Carbohydrates on Mood and Behavior," *Nutrition Reviews Supplement* 44 (May 1986): 51–60.

24. Bonnie Spring et al., *Journal of Psychiatric Research* 17: (1982/83): 155.

25. Craig, "Acute Effects of Meals," 165.

26. Ronald Prinz and David Riddle, "Associations Between Nutrition and Behavior in Five Year Old Children," *Nutrition Reviews Supplement* 44 (May 1986): 151–57.

27. C. Keith Conners, "Carbohydrates and Sucrose: Psychological, Cognitive and Behavioral Effects" (Paper presented at the 95th Annual Meeting of the American Psychological Association, New York, 31 August 1987).

28. Ibid.

29. Judith Rapoport, "Diet and Hyperactivity," *Nutrition Reviews Supplement* 44 (May 1986): 158–62.

30. Arthur Winter and Ruth Winter, *Build Your Brain Power* (New York: St. Martin's Press, 1986), 133.

31. S. J. Schoenthaler, *International Journal of Biosocial Research* 5: 79–87.

32. Winter and Winter, *Brain Power,* 133.

33. S. J. Schoenthaler, *Biosocial Research,* 79–87.

34. Bonnie Spring, "Carbohydrate Craving: Clinical Implications" (Paper presented at the 94th Annual Meeting of the American Psychological Association, Washington, D. C., 23 August 1986).

35. Judith Wurtman, "Carbohydrate Craving in Obesity" (Paper presented at the 94th Annual Meeting of the American Psychological Association, Washington, D.C., 23 August 1986).

36. Ibid.

37. Neal Grunberg and Deborah Bowen, "Carbohydrate Craving in Bulimic Individuals" (Paper presented at the 94th Annual Meeting of the American Psychological Association, Washington, D.C., 23 August 1986).

38. Ibid.

39. Norman E. Rosenthal et al., "Carbohydrate and Protein Meals: Acute Effects on Mood and Performance" (Paper presented at the 94th Annual Meeting of the American Psychological Association, Washington, D.C., 23 August 1986).

40. June Chiodo, "Carbohydrate Craving in Bulimic Individuals" (Paper presented at the 94th Annual Meeting of the American Psychological Association, Washington, D. C., 23 August 1986.

41. Phyllis Crapo, "Theory vs. Fact: Glycemic Response to Food," *Nutrition Today* 19 (2): 6–12.

42. Ibid.

43. Gina Kolata, "Diabetics Should Lose

Weight, Avoid Diet Fads," *Science,* 9 January 1987, 235.

44. Gina Kolata, "High-Carbohydrate Diets Questioned," *Science,* 9 January 1987, 164.

45. Chris Lecos, "Sugar: How Sweet It Is—And Isn't," *FDA Consumer,* February 1980, 21–23.

46. R. E. Hodges and W. H. Krehl, "The Role of Carbohydrates in Lipid Metabolism," *American Journal of Clinical Nutrition* 17 (1965): 334–46.

47. Hans Fisher and Eugene Boe, *The Rutgers Guide to Lowering Your Cholesterol* (New Brunswick, N.J.: Rutgers University Press, 1985), 85.

CHAPTER 5.

Using Food to Protect Your Brain Against Stroke and Other Damage

1. "Regulation of Water and Sodium Homeostatus," in *Merck Manual,* 14th ed., ed. Robert Berkow (Rahway, N.J.: Merck, 1982), 922–24.

2. Food and Drug Administration, "Preliminary Data: FY 77 Selected Minerals in Food Survey / Total Diet Studies," Department of Health, Education and Welfare, Washington, D.C., 1978.

3. *FDA Consumer,* October 1981, Health and Human Services pub. no. FDA 82–2158.

4. A. M. Osterfeld, "A Review of Stroke Epidemiology," *Epidemiological Review* 2 (1980): 136–52; and Kay-Tee Khaw and Elizabeth Barrett-Connor, "Dietary Potassium and Stroke-Associated Mortality," *New England Journal of Medicine* 316 (5): 235–36.

5. "Lite-Line Snacks Trim Fat But Not Taste," *Consumer Reports,* March 1985, 127.

6. L. K Dahlet, "Salt and Hypertension," *American Journal of Clinical Nutrition* 25 (1972):231–44.

7. Myron Weinberger, Judith Miller, et al., "Genetic Markers for Salt Sensitivity" (Paper presented at the 59th Scientific Sessions of the American Heart Association, Dallas, 19 November 1986).

8. "How Stress Causes High Blood Pressure," *Science News,* 23 April 1983, 261.

9. Rose Stamler et al., "Nutritional Therapy for High Blood Pressure: Final Report of a Four Year Randomized Controlled Trial—The Hypertension Control Program," *Journal of the American Medical Association* 257 (11): 1484–91.

10. S. M. Grundy, "Comparison of Monounsaturated Fatty Acids and Carbohydrates for Lowering Plasma Cholesterol," *New England Journal of Medicine* 314 (12): 745–48.

11. Ruth Winter, *Cancer Causing Agents: A Preventive Guide,* (New York: Crown, 1979), 99.

12. A. Keys, "Lowering Plasma Cholesterol by Diet," *New England Journal of Medicine* 315 (9): 585.

13. American Heart Association, *Cardiovascular Research Report,* no. 20 (Dallas: American Heart Association, 1985), 6.

14. Ann Williams, "Garlic Yields Anti-Clotting Compound," *Cardiovascular Research Report,* no. 20 (Dallas: American Heart Association, (1985), 7.

15. Ibid.

16. Edward Knapp, "Fish Oil Concentrate Produces Beneficial Effects" (Paper presented at the 58th Scientific Sessions of the American Heart Association, Washington D.C., 12 November 1985).

17. Ibid.

CHAPTER 6.

The Allergy/Brain/Behavior Connection

1. Michael Kaliner, "Allergy and Infectious Diseases," U.S. Department of Health and Human Services, National Institutes of Health pub. no. 81–1948, (1981).

2. American Academy of Allergy and Immunology, "Adverse Reactions to Foods," National Institutes of Health pub. no. 84–2442 (July 1984).

3. Richard Thompson, "Food Allergies: Separating Fact from 'Hype,' " *FDA Consumer,* June 1986, 25–26.

4. Academy of Allergy and Immunology, "Adverse Reactions to Foods."

5. "Pain in the Head," *Harvard Medical School Health Letter* 5 (2): 1–3.

6. Thompson, "Food Allergies," 25–26.

7. Joan Arehart-Treichel, "Migraines: Unmasking the Causes," *Science News,* 11 October 1980, 237.

8. "Making Migraines Amine-able," *Medical World News,* 31 October 1969.

9. W. R. Shannon, *American Journal of Diseases of Children* 24 (1922): 89–94.

10. F. Speer, "Allergic Tension Fatigue in Children," *Annals of Allergy* 12 (1954): 168–171.

11. B. F. Feingold, *Why Your Child is Hyperactive* (New York: Random House, 1975).

12. E. B. Nasr et al., "Concordance of Atopic and Affective Disorders," *Journal of Affective Disorders* 3 (1981): 291; and H. J. Ossofsky, "Affective and Atopic Disorders and Cyclic AMP," *Comparative Psychiatry* 17 (1976): 335.

13. Academy of Allergy and Immunology, "Adverse Reactions to Foods," 72–74.

14. H. G. Kinnell et al., "Food Antibodies in Schizophrenia," *Psychological Medicine* 12 (1982):85–89.

15. "Childhood Autism Linked to Brain Allergy," *Science News,* 27 November 1982, 340.

16. Benjamin Wolozin et al., "A Neuronal Antigen in the Brains of Alzheimer Patients," *Science,* 2 May 1986, 648–50.

17. John Crayton, "Adverse Reactions to Foods: Relevance to Psychiatric Disorders," *Journal of Allergy and Clinical Immunology* 78 (July 1986): 243–47.

CHAPTER 7.
Food and Drug Interactions

1. D. A. Roe, "Diet-Drug Interactions and Incompatibilities," in *Nutrient and Drug Interactions,* ed. N. Hathcock and J. Coon (New York: Academic Press, 1978), 319–45.

2. M. A. Diamond et al., "Treatment of Idiopathic Postural Hypertension with Oral Tyramine and Monoamine Oxidase Inhibitor," *Journal of Clinical Research* 17: 237.

3. Attallah Kappas, personal communication with authors, 13 April 1985.

4. Ibid.

5. Karl Anderson, personal communication with authors, 25 February 1987.

6. Kappas, personal communication.

7. Ruth Winter, interview with Attallah Kappas, *Register and Tribune Syndicate,* 13 February 1983.

8. "Drugs and the Elderly," *Medical Forum,* June 1984, 3–4.

9. Anderson, personal communication.

10. Ibid.

11. Glenn B. Raiczyk and John Pinto, "Troublesome Combinations and Susceptible Patients," *Consultant,* July 1986, 85–105.

12. J. D. O'Keefe and V. Marx, "Lunch-Time Gin and Tonic: A Cause of Reactive Hypoglycemia," *Lancet 1* (1977): 1286–87.

13. "Drinking and Driving: How Much Is Too Much?" *Harvard Medical School Health Letter,* 8 (4): 6.

14. P. Wainwright et al., "Combined Effects of Moderate Ethanol Consumption and a Low-Protein Diet During Gestation on Brain Development in BALB/c Mice," *Experimental Neurology* 90 (2): 422–33.

15. Brian L. G. Morgan, *Food and Drug Interaction Guide* (New York: Simon and Schuster, 1986), 271.

16. Raiczyk and Pinto, "Troublesome Combinations and Susceptible Patients," 85–105.

CHAPTER 8.
Have You Eaten Any Neurotoxins Lately?

1. Jane Hersey, personal communication with authors, 8 May 1987.

2. Bernard Weiss et al., "Behavioral Response to Artificial Colors," *Science,* 8 March 1980, 1487–89.

3. J. Egger et al., "Controlled Trial of Oligoantigenic Treatment in The Hyperkinetic Syndrome," *Lancet,* 9 March 1985, 540–44.

4. George Augustine, Jr., and Herbert Levitan, "Neurotransmitter Release from a Vertebrate Neuromuscular Synapse Af-

fected by a Food Dye," *Science,* 28 March 1980, 1489–90.

5. *Food Product Development,* December 1980: 36–40.

6. Charles Vorhees and R. E. Butcher, *Developmental Toxicology,* ed. K. Snell (London: Croom Helm, 1982), 247–98.

7. Bernard Weiss, "Food Additives and Environmental Chemicals as Sources of Childhood Behavior Disorders," *Journal of the American Academy of Child Psychiatry* 21 (March 1982): 144–152.

8. George Wagner, personal communication with authors, 29 April 1987.

9. Bernard Weiss, personal communication with authors, 29 April 1987.

10. Peter Spencer "Environmental Hypothesis for Brain Diseases," *Science* 31 July 1987, 517.

11. Harold Schmeck, Jr., "Significance Seen in a Guam Disease," *New York Times* 31 July 1987, B20.

12. Weiss, personal communication.

13. American Academy of Pediatrics, press release, 5 March 1987.

14. "Trace Metals Leave More than Trace Effects," *Science News,* 16 June 1984, 373.

15. Ibid.

16. National Institutes of Health, press packet, December 1986.

17. "Alzheimer's Research Aims at Aluminum," *Advertising Age,* 23 June 1986, 12.

18. Walter Sullivan, "Metal's Link to Alzheimer's Studied," *New York Times,* 2 May 1987, 27.

19. Ralph M. Garruto et al., "Intraneuronal Co-Localization of Silicon with Calcium and Aluminum in Amyotrophic Lateral Sclerosis and Parkinsonism with Dementia of Guam," *New England Journal of Medicine* 315 (11 September 1986).

20. Annabel Hecht, "Searching for Clues to Alzheimer's Disease," *FDA Consumer,* November 1985, 23–24.

21. "Alcohol Found to Impair Pilots Hours Later," *New York Times,* 7 December 1986, 39.

22. Ibid.

23. Louis Goldfrank, "Ask Me About Alcohol Withdrawal," *Emergency Medicine,* 30 September 1986, 24–28.

24. "Heavy Drinking Shrinks The Brain," Reuters (London), 8 December 1984.

25. "The Alcoholic's Shrinking Brain," *Science News,* 7 February 1981, 87.

26. Constance Holden, "Alcoholism and the Medical Cost Crunch," *Science,* 6 March 1987, 132–33.

27. *Morbidity and Mortality Weekly Report,* 14 November 1986, 703.

28. Jaswinder S. Gill et al., "Stroke and Alcohol Consumption," *New England Journal of Medicine* 315 (17): 1041–50.

29. Ibid.

30. R. P. Donahue et al., "Alcohol and Hemorrhagic Stroke," *Journal of the American Medical Association* 255: 2311–14; and M. Hillbon and M. Kast, "Does Alcohol Intoxication Precipitate Aneurysmal Hemorrhage?" *Journal of Neurology and Psychiatry* 44 (1981): 523–26.

31. William Hazle, "Diagnosis of Drug and Alcohol Addiction" (Paper presented at Alcohol Studies Program, University of California at Santa Cruz, 20 September 1987.

32. National Institute on Alcohol Abuse and Alcoholism, "Alcohol Health and Research World," U.S. Department of Health and Human Services, pub. no. ADM 85–151 (1985), 44.

33. Ibid.

34. Ibid., 27.

35. Ibid.

36. Roger Maickel, "Pituitary Stress / Alcoholism Key" (Paper presented at the 25th Annual Meeting of The American College of Neuropharmacology, Washington, D. C., 11 December 1986).

37. Ibid.

38. U.S. Department of Health and Human Services, *Phobias and Panic,* DHHS pub. no. ADM 86–1472 (1986), 20.

39. Thomas Uhde, "Biological Issues in Panic" (Paper presented at National Conference on Phobias and Related Anxiety Disorders, New York, 17 October 1986).

40. Carol Mithers, "The Caffeine, Coffee,

Cola and Chocolate Debate," *Self,* August 1979, 10.

41. Richard Gilbert, "Caffeine: History, Habits and Health," *The Journal of the Addiction Research Foundation* (Ontario) 1 October 1984, 5.

42. P. W. Curatolo and D. Robertson, "The Health Consequences of Caffeine," *Annals of Internal Medicine* 98 (5): 641–53.

43. Morris A. Shorofsky and Norman Lamm, *New York State Journal of Medicine,* February 1977; and Gilbert, "Caffeine," 528.

44. Phoenix (Arizona) Department of Health Services, *Decision on Petition for Tolerance Regulation and Embargo in Arizona of Carbonated Beverages and Carbonated Beverage Syrup Bases Containing Aspartame,* 7 March 1984.

45. American Council on Scientific Affairs, "Aspartame: Review of Safety Issues," *Journal of the American Medical Association* 254 (1985): 400–02.

46. "Aspartame Hearings Rejected," *American Medical News,* 12 December 1986, 21.

47. "Aspartame Critics Persist: Recommend Avoidance During Pregnancy," *Medical World News,* 27 February 1984, 23–24.

48. Ibid.

49. Dennis Choi et al., "Glutamate Neurotoxicity in Cortical Cell Culture," *Journal of Neuroscience* 7 (2): 357–68.

50. Dennis Choi, "Ionic Dependence of Glutamate Neurotoxicity," *Journal of Neuroscience* 7 (2): 369–79.

51. W. F. Maragos et al., "Co-Localization of Congo Red-Stained Neurofibrillary Tangles in Glutamate Immunoreactive Neurons in the Hippocampus" (Paper presented at the 16th Annual Meeting of the Society for Neuroscience, Washington, D.C., November 1986).

52. Erik Eckolm, "Monosodium Glutamate Still a Mystery," *New York Times,* 23 April 1986.

53. Ruth Winter, *A Consumer's Dictionary of Food Additives* (New York: Crown, 1984), 167.

54. Thomas J. Sobotka, "The Regulatory Perspective of Diet-Behavior Relationships," *Nutrition Reviews Supplement* 44 (May 1986): 241–43.

55. Thomas J. Sobotka, personal communication with authors, 5 May 1987.

56. Statistics were supplied by U.S. Food and Drug Administration spokesperson, 5 May 1987.

57. *Food Product Development,* December 1980: 36–40.

58. Thomas J. Sobotka, personal communication with authors, 5 May 1987.

59. Ibid.

60. Ibid.

61. Sobotka, "Diet-Behavior Relationships," 241.

62. L. Barry Goss, personal communication with authors, 29 April 1987.

63. Ibid.

64. Ibid.; and L. Barry Goss and Thomas D. Sabourin, "Utilization of Alternative Species for Toxicity Testing: An Overview," *Journal of Applied Toxicology* 5 (4): 193–219.

65. Pennington Associates, "CIIT, Founded by Chemical Industry, is a Unique Toxicology Research Facility" (Pennington Associates, Raleigh, N.C.), 29 April 1987, 1–14.

66. Ibid.

67. Hugh A. Tilson, personal communication with authors, 3 May 1987.

CHAPTER 9.
Building a Child's Brain Power with Food

1. "Fetal Distress from Something Mother Ate," *Emergency Medicine,* 15 April 1985, 87.

2. J. A. Miller, "Brain Already Busy While in the Womb," *Science News,* 20 October 1984.

3. Ibid.

4. R. Balazs et al., *Human Growth,* vol. 3, *Neurobiology and Nutrition,* ed. F. Falkner and J. M. Tanner (New York: Plenum Press, 1979), 415–80.

5. "Nutrition and Behavior," *Dairy Council Digest* 50 (5).

6. U.S. Department of Health and

Human Services, Public Health Service, Alcohol Drug Abuse and Mental Health Administration, "The Neuroscience of Mental Health, a Report on Neuroscience Research from Panels of Scientists Representative of Contributing Disciplines," 1985, p. 96.

7. Herman Baker, personal communication with authors, January 1987.

8. Harold Sandstead, "Nutrition and Brain Function: Trace Elements," *Nutrition Reviews Supplement* (May 1986): 37–41.

9. Ibid.

10. Ibid.

11. Carl C. Pfeiffer and Eric Braverman, "Zinc, the Brain and Behavior," *Biological Psychiatry* 17 (4): 513–19.

12. Sandstead, "Nutrition and Brain Function," 37–41.

13. M. W. Miller, "The Time of Origin of Neurons in Rat Motor Cortex in Experimental Fetal Alcohol Syndrome," (Paper presented at the 16th Annual Meeting of the Society for Neuroscience, Washington, D.C., November 1986).

14. "Study Notes Alcohol Use Can Affect Birth Weight," *American Medical News,* 19 September 1986, 7.

15. "Booze and Pregnancy: The Pickled Brain," *Science News,* 17 January 1980.

16. Statement of The American Academy of Pediatrics, 1 October 1986.

17. B. Frieder and V. E. Grimm, "Prenatal Caffeine Causes Long Lasting Behavioral and Neurochemical Changes," (Paper presented at the 16th Annual Meeting of the Society for Neuroscience, Washington, D.C., November 1986).

18. U.S. Department of Health and Human Services, "The Neural Basis of Psychopathology: The Neuroscience of Mental Health," DHHS Pub. no. 9 (1985), 96–97.

19. Marvin Eiger and Sally Wendkos Olds, *The Complete Book of Breast Feeding* (New York: Workman, 1987), 59–60.

20. Dori Stehlin, "Good Nutrition for Breast Feeding Mothers," *FDA Consumer,* December 1986 to January 1987, 33–36.

21. *National Research Council, Bulletin* no. 123 (Washington, D.C.: National Research Council of the National Academy of Sciences, 1950).

22. Eiger and Olds, *Complete Book of Breast Feeding.*

23. "New View on Feeding Babies," *Medical Forum,* August 1982.

24. S. A. Richardson, H. G. Birch and M. E. Hertzig, *American Journal of Mental Deficiency* 77 (1973): 623.

25. Z. A. Stein et al., *Famine and Human Development: The Dutch Hunger Winter of 1944–45* (New York: Oxford University Press, 1975).

26. Merrill Read, "Malnutrition and Behavior," *Applied Research in Mental Retardation* 3 (1982): 279–91.

27. J. Cravito, "Nutrition, Stimulation, Mental Development and Learning," *Nutrition Today,* September/October 1981, 4–15.

28. Ibid.

29. Ibid.

30. Derek Bryce-Smith "Environmental Chemical Influences on Behavior, Personality and Mentation," *International Journal of Biosocial Research* 8 (2): 115–47.

31. Ellen Hale, "Good Nutrition for Your Growing Child," *FDA Consumer,* April 1987, 21.

32. Jane Brody, "Parents' Attitudes Toward Diet Can Contribute to Obesity in Children and Adolescents," *New York Times,* 27 May 1987, C7.

33. Hale, "Good Nutrition for Your Child," 21.

34. A. M. Mauer and H. S. Dweck, "Toward A Prudent Diet For Children," *Pediatrics* 71(1): 78–79.

35. Michael Pugliese and Fima Lifshitz, "Parents' Misconceptions on Diet, Health Can Delay Growth of Their Infants," news release, American Academy of Pediatrics, 5 August 1987.

36. Hale "Good Nutrition for Your Child," 26.

37. National Institute of Child Health and Human Development, workshop, Bethesda, Md., 10–11 March 1986.

38. Hale, "Good Nutrition for Your Child," 23.

39. Gina Kolata, "Obese Children: A

Growing Problem," *Science,* 4 April 1986.

40. A. W. Logue, *The Psychology of Eating and Drinking* (New York: Freeman, 1986), 99.

41. R. J. Prinz et al., *Journal of Consulting Clinical Psychology* 48 (1980): 760–69.

42. D. Behar et al., "Sugar Challenge Testing with Children Considered Behaviorally 'Sugar Reactive,' " *Nutritional Behavior* 1 (1984): 279–88.

43. C. K. Conners and A. G. Blouin, *Research Strategies for Assessing the Behavioral Effects of Foods and Nutrients* (Cambridge: MIT Press, 1982), 132–44.

44. Judith Rapoport, "Diet and Hyperactivity," *Nutrition Reviews Supplement* (May 1986): 158–62.

45. Rois Pertz and Lillian Putnam, "The Reading Teacher," 35 (March 1982): 702–06.

46. Ibid.

47. Ibid.

48. Stephen Schoenthaler et al., "The Impact of Low Food Additive and Sucrose Diet on Academic Performance in 803 New York City Public Schools," *International Journal of Biosocial Research* 8 (2): 185–95.

49. Stephen Schoenthaler et al., "The Testing of Various Hypotheses as Explanations for the Gains in National Test Scores in the 1978–1983 New York City Nutrition Policy Modification Project," *International Journal of Biosocial Research* 8 (2): 198–99.

50. Ibid.

51. W. Weidman et al., "American Heart Association Committee Report: Diet in the Healthy Child," *Circulation* 67 (June 1983): 1411–13A.

CHAPTER 10.

Maintaining and Improving Adult Brain Power Through Food

1. Edward L. Schneider et al., "Recommended Dietary Allowances and the Health of the Elderly," *New England Journal of Medicine* 314, 16 January 1986: 157–60.

2. Chris Lecos, "Diet and the Elderly: Research Points to Some Special Needs," *FDA Consumer,* October 1984, 27–29.

3. Chris Lecos, "Diet and the Elderly," *FDA Consumer,* September 1984, 23–25.

4. A. J. Gelenberg, J. C. Dollere-Wojcik, and J. H. Growdon, "Choline and Lecithin in the Treatment of Tardive Dyskinesia: Preliminary Results from a Pilot Study," *American Journal of Psychiatry* 136: 772–76.

5. Robert Butler, *Nutrition in the 1980s: Constraints on Our Knowledge* (New York: Alan Liss, Inc., 1981), 207–17.

6. James F. Flood, Gary Smith, and John Morley, "Modulation of Memory Processing by Cholecystokinin: Dependence on the Vagus Nerve," *Science,* 15 May 1987, 832–34.

7. Hoffman-La Roche, Inc., "An Introduction to Free Radicals," *Vitamin Nutrition Information Service Backgrounder"* 1 (March 1986).

8. Purdue University, "Purdue Tests Natural Antioxidants," Special report, 12 May 1986, p. 1.

9. Ibid.

10. Larry Christensen, "Hypoglycemia: Implications and Suggestions for Research," *Journal of Orthomolecular Psychiatry* 10 (2): 77–92; and Carl Pfeiffer, "Psychiatric Hospital vs. Brain Bio Center in Diagnosis of Biochemical Imbalances," *Journal of Orthomolecular Psychiatry* 5 (1): 28–34.

11. Rockefeller University, *Research Profiles,* Spring 1987, 1–4

12. Ibid.

13. Ibid.

14. P. F. Aravich et al., "High Fat, High Sucrose Feeding and Exercise: Relationship to Vasopressin and Oxytocin in the Rat" (Paper presented at the 16th Annual Meeting of the Society for Neruoscience, Washington, D. C., November 1986).

15. R. Woo and F. Pi-Sunyer, "Effect of Increased Physical Activity on Voluntary Intake in Lean Women," *Metabolism* 34 (September 1985): 836–41.

16. *Tufts University Diet and Nutrition Letter* 3 (12): 6.

17. Robert Matz "Obesity: An Eclectic Review", *Hospital Practice,* 15 February 1987, 152.

CHAPTER 11.
Hunger, Appetite, and Your Brain

1. Ruth Winter, "Appetite Control—The Secret Is at the Base of Your Brain," *Science Digest,* October 1980, 8–13.

2. A. W. Heatherington and S. W. Ranson, "Hypothalamic Lesions and Adiposity in the Rat," *Anatomical Record* 78(1940): 149–72.

3. M. L. Caldwell et al., "A Clinical Note on Food Preference of Individuals with Prader-Willi Syndrome," *Journal of Mental Deficiency Research* 27(1):45–49.

4. B. K. Arnand and J. R. Brobeck, "Localization of the Feeding Center in the Hypothalamus of the Rat," *Proceedings of the Society for Experimental Biology and Medicine* 77(1951):323–24.

5. Stellar, "The Physiology of Motivation," *Psychological Review* 61(1954):5–22.

6. A. W. Logue, *The Psychology of Eating and Drinking* (New York: Freeman, 1986), 19.

7. J. Mayer, "The Glucostatic Theory of Regulation of Food Intake and the Problem of Obesity," *Bulletin of the New England Medical Center* 14(1952):43–49.

8. John E. Morley et al., "Neuropeptides and Appetite: Contribution of Neuropharmacological Modeling," *Federation Proceedings* 43(14):2903–07.

9. "Hypothalamic Link with GI Tract," *Science News,* 13 September 1980, 165.

10. S. F. Leibowitz and C. Rossakis, *Neuropharmacology* 17:691–702.

11. Ibid.

12. John E. Blundell, "Serotonin Manipulations and the Structure of Feeding Behavior, in *Appetite* (London: Academic Press, 1986), 39–56.

13. Allen S. Levine, and John Morley, "The Shortening Pathways to Appetite Control," *Nutrition Today,* January/February 1983, 6–9.

14. Mark Friedman, "New Perspectives on the Metabolic Basis of Hunger and Satiety," *Contemporary Nutrition* 7 (May 1982).

15. Ibid.

16. Harry Kissileff, "Satiety," *Journal of Dentistry for Children* S2(5): 386–89.

17. Ibid.

18. Ibid.

19. Charles Pollak, interview with authors, Cornell Medical Center, Westchester, N.Y., November 1986.

20. B. Andersson and S. M. McCann, "Drinking, Antidiuresis and Milk Ejection from Electrical Stimulation Within the Hypothalamus of the Goat," *Acta Physiologica Scandinavica* 35(1955):191–201.

21. Ibid.

22. Logue, *Psychology of Eating and Drinking,* 39.

23. W. B. Cannon, "The Physiological Basis of Thirst," in *The Foundations of Experimental Psychology,* ed. C. Murchison (Worcester, Mass.: Clark University Press, 1929).

24. Logue, *Psychology of Eating and Drinking,* 43.

25. Ibid.

26. Jan Oswald and K. Adam, "Rhythmic Raiding of Refrigerator Related to Rapid Eye Movements Sleep," *British Medical Journal* (1986): 292–99.

27. J. T. Metz et al., "Effect of Electrical Stimulation to the Human Brain (VMH) on Regional Cerebral Metabolism" (Paper presented at the 16th Annual Meeting of the Society for Neuroscience, Washington, D.C., November 1986.

28. Dixie Farley, "Eating Disorders: When Thinness Becomes an Obsession," *FDA Consumer,* May 1986, 20–22.

29. Renfrew Center (Philadelphia) Fact Sheet on Bulimia, 1986.

30. David B. Herzog and Paul Copeland, "Eating Disorders" *New England Journal of Medicine* 313 (5): 295–303.

31. Walter Kaye et al., "Elevated Cerebrospinal Fluid Levels of Immunoreactive Corticotropin-Releasing Hormone in Anorexia Nervosa," *Journal of Clinical Endocrinology and Metabolism* 64 (2):203–07.

32. Sarah Leibowitz, personal communication with authors, 7 April 1987.

33. Ibid.

34. Ibid.

35. Ibid.

36. National Institutes of Health, Consensus Development Conference, "Health Implications of Obesity," 5 (9).

37. "Just Looking at Food Can Make Fat People Fatter," *ADAMHA News,* 2 February 1980, 3.

38. Ibid.

CHAPTER 12.
Choices—Why You Eat What You Do

1. Erik Eckholm, "Children and Food: How Eating Habits Are Formed," *International Herald Tribune,* 29 July 1985, 16.

2. Richard Rivlin, "The Use of Hormones in the Treatment of Obesity," *Current Concepts in Nutrition* 3 (1975): 151–62.

3. Susan Schiffman, "Taste and Smell in Disease," *New England Journal of Medicine* 308 (22): 1337.

4. Susan Schiffman "Mechanisms of Disease," *New England Journal of Medicine* 308 (22): 1339.

5. Maura Rhodes, "Yum and Yuck: When Food Cravings and Aversions Tell You About Your Health," *Self,* October 1986, 184–85.

6. Sarah Leibowitz, interview with authors, 23 April 1987.

7. John Blundell, "Problems and Processes Underlying the Control of Food Selection and Nutrient Intake," *Nutrition and the Brain,* vol. 6, ed. R. J. and J. J. Wurtman, (New York: Raven Press, 1983), 164.

8. C. M. Davis, "Self Selection of Diet by Newly Weaned Infants," *American Journal of Diseases of Children* 36 (1928): 651–79.

9. "Shaping Budding Tastes," *Tufts University Diet and Nutrition Letter* 5 (2): 17–19.

10. Bertram Gordon, "Why We Choose the Foods We Do," *Nutrition Today* 18 (March/April 1983): 17–19.

11. Ibid.

12. Ibid.

13. Susan Schiffman, "The Use of Flavor to Enhance Efficacy of Reducing Diets," *Hospital Practice,* 15 July 1986, 44H–44R.

14. Ibid.

15. "Dieters Binge Away: This Chocolate Treat is Lighter than Air," *Advertising Age,* 9 March 1987, 55.

16. Neil Grunberg et al., "The Importance of Sweet Taste and Caloric Content: The Effects of Nicotine on Specific Food Consumption," *Pharmacology* 87 (1985): 198–203.

17. Jeanine Louis-Sylvestre, "Meal Size: Role of Reflexly Induced Insulin Release," *Journal of the Autonomic Nervous System* 10 (January 1984): 317–24.

18. U.S. Department of Health, Education, and Welfare, "Nutrition and Aging," DHEW pub. no. NIH 78–1409 (1978).

19. "Shaping Budding Tastes," 17–19.

20. David Kurtz and Louis Boone, *Marketing,* 3d ed. (Chicago: Dryden, 1987), 14.

CHAPTER 13.
Use Your Brain to Choose Your Diet

1. Trish Hall, "What Americans Eat Hasn't Changed Much Despite Healthy Image," *Wall Street Journal,* 12 Sept 1985, pp. 1 and 20.

2. *Tufts University Diet & Nutrition Letter* (12):3.

3. A. S. Levine, T. P. Labuza, and J. E. Morley, "Food Technology: A Primer for Physicians," *New England Journal of Medicine* 312 (10): 628–33.

Glossary

Acetylcholine. A neurotransmitter that is released by nerve cells and acts on either other nerve cells or muscles and organs throughout the body. This neurotransmitter is believed to be involved in memory function.

ACTH. Adrenocorticotropic hormone, a hormone controller.

Action potential. An electric burst that travels the length of the nerve cell and causes the release of a neurotransmitter.

Adrenal gland. About the size of a grape, your two adrenal glands lie on top of each of your kidneys. Each adrenal gland has two parts. The first part is the medulla, which produces epinephrine and norepinephrine, two hormones that play a part in controlling your heart rate and blood pressure. Signals from your brain stimulate production of these hormones. The second part is the adrenal cortex, which produces three groups of steroid hormones. The hormones in one group control the levels of various chemicals in your body. For example, they prevent the loss of too much sodium and water into the urine. Aldosterone is the most important hormone in this group. The hormones in the second group have a number of functions. One is to help convert carbohydrates, or starches, into energy-providing glycogen in your liver. Hydrocortisone is the main hormone in this group. The third group consists of the male hormone androgen and the female hormones estrogen and progesterone.

Agonist. A drug, hormone, or neurotransmitter that binds to a receptor site and triggers a response.

Alzheimer's disease. A deterioration of the brain with severe memory impairment.

Amino acids. Building blocks of proteins and neurotransmitters.

Angiotensin. A powerful elevator of blood pressure, angiotensin is produced by the action of renin, an enzyme made in the kidney. All of the components of the renin-angiotensin system have been found in the brain, and there are indications that they are part of the brain's mechanism for regulating blood pressure as well as for telling you when you should or should not drink fluid.

Antagonist. A drug, hormone, or neurotransmitter that blocks a response from a receptor site.

Anticholinergic. The blocking of acetylcholine receptors, which results in the inhibition of nerve impulse transmission.

Arteriosclerosis. Commonly known as "hardening of the arteries," arteriosclerosis includes a variety of conditions that cause the artery walls to thicken and lose elasticity.

Aspartic acid. A nonessential amino acid.

259

Atherosclerosis. A form of arteriosclerosis. The inner layers of the artery walls are made thick and irregular by deposits of a fatty substance. The internal channel of the arteries becomes narrowed, reducing blood supply.

Autonomic nervous system. The division of the nervous system that regulates the involuntary vital functions, such as the activity of the heart and breathing.

Axon. The principal fiber of a nerve.

Calcium messenger system. As calcium ions increase in the cell, a specific receptor protein, calmodulin, interacts with other proteins to initiate cell responses such as smooth muscle contraction. The calcium messenger system is believed to play a part in learning.

Calmodulin. *See* Calcium messenger system

Catecholamines. A group of self-made chemicals such as neurotransmitters and hormones, which can be made synthetically. Among the major catecholamines are dopamine, norepinepherine, and epinepherine. The catecholamines are involved in the regulation of blood pressure, heart rate, muscle tone, metabolism, and central nervous system function.

CCK. *See* Cholecystokinin

Cerebral thrombosis. Formation of a blood clot in a vessel leading to the brain.

Cerebral vascular accident. Apoplexy, or stroke, an impeded blood supply to part of the brain.

Cholecystokinin (CCK). A hormone produced by the small intestine during the movement of food from the stomach into the intestine. CCK causes the contraction of the gall bladder, thus releasing bile into the small intestine, where the enzymes and other components of bile aid digestion. This hormone has also been found in the brain and may help to stop eating.

Choline. Found in most animal tissues, either free or in combinations such as lecithin or acetylcholine. Choline is being actively studied for its effects on brain neurotransmission and memory.

Cholinesterase. The enzyme that processes the neurotransmitter acetylcholine. There is a great deal of scientific interest in this enzyme, particularly in the study of Alzheimer's disease (*See* Alzheimer's disease), because it is believed to be involved in poor memory function.

Corticotropin-releasing factor (CRF). A neurotransmitter involved in appetite and stress reactions.

CRF. *See* Corticotropin-releasing factor

Cysteine. A nonessential amino acid.

Cystine. A product of cysteine, produced by oxidation and sometimes found in urine. Used to treat brittle nails.

Dendrites. Spiderlike projections from the cell body that receive and send messages between nerve cells.

Diuretic. A drug that promotes the excretion of urine.

Dopamine. 3-hydroxytyramine—an intermediate in tyrosine metabolism and the precursor of norepinepherine and epinepherine. Dopamine is involved in movement and mood.

Endorphins. Self-made tranquilizers and pain killers. Each endorphin is composed of a chain of amino acids and acts on the nervous system to reduce pain.

Enkephalins. Self-made pain killers to which endorphins belong.

Epinepherine. Adrenaline. The major hormone of the adrenal gland, epinepherine increases heart rate and contractions, vasoconstriction or vasodilation, relaxation of the muscles in the lungs and of smooth muscles in the intestines and the processing of sugar and fat.

GABA. *See* Gamma-aminobutyric acid.

Gamma-aminobutyric acid (GABA). A compound, found in high concentrations in the brain, that functions as an inhibitory neurotransmitter.

GHRH. *See* Growth hormone-releasing hormone

Glucagon. A neurotransmitter involved in glucose metabolism and hunger.

Glutamic acid. A nonessential amino acid.

Glycine. A nonessential amino acid, usually derived from gelatin.

Growth hormone-releasing hormone (GHRH). A hormone that stimulates the release of sex hormones.

Hypoglycemia. Low blood sugar—the opposite of diabetes.

Hypothalamus. Brain control area involved in emotions, movement, and eating. Less than the size of a peanut and weighing a quarter of an ounce, this small area deep within the brain also oversees appetite, blood pressure, sexual behavior, sleep, and emotions, and sends orders to the pituitary gland.

LHRH. *See* Luteinizing hormone-releasing hormone

Luteinizing hormone-releasing hormone (LHRH). A hormone that helps regulate sex hormones.

Monamine. Containing one amine group.

Monoamine oxidase inhibitors (MAOI's). A group of drugs that is used in the treatment of depression and that elevates the level of neurotransmitters by preventing their destruction by enzymes.

Neuron. The basic nerve cell of the central nervous system, containing a nucleus within the cell body, an axon (a trunklike projection containing neurotransmitters), and dendrites (spiderlike projections that send and receive messages).

Neuropeptide Y. A neurotransmitter believed to cause carbohydrate craving.

Neurotensin. A peptide of thirteen amino acid derivatives that helps regulate blood sugar by its effects on a number of hormones, including insulin and glucagon. It is also thought to play a part in pain suppression.

Neurotransmitters. Molecules that carry chemical messages between nerve cells. Neurotransmitters are released from a nerve cell, diffuse across the minute distance between two nerve cells (synaptic cleft), and bind to a receptor at another nerve site.

Nerve growth factor (NGF). Believed to maintain and repair nerves in the brain.

NGF. *See* Nerve growth factor

Norepinephrine. Noradrenaline, a hormone released by the adrenal gland, possessing the ability to stimulate, as does epinephrine, but with minimal inhibitatory effects. It has little effect on the lungs' smooth muscles and metabolic processes and differs from epinephrine in its effect on the heart and blood vessels.

Oxytocin. A pituitary hormone that stimulates muscle contraction.

Parasympathetic nervous system. A group of nerve fibers that leave the brain and spinal cord and extend to nerve cell clusters (ganglia) at specific sites. From there they are distributed to blood vessels, glands, and other internal organs. Parasympathetic nerves are involved in the heart rate, stimulating digestion, and contracting bronchioles in the lungs, pupils in the eyes, and the esophagus. The parasympathetic nervous system works in conjunction with the sympathetic nervous system (*see* Sympathetic nervous system).

Parathyroid gland. On the four corners of the thyroid gland (*see* Thyroid gland), these pearl-sized glands produce parathyroid hormones, which work with calcitonin from the thyroid gland to control calcium in the blood. Calcium not only has a role in developing bones and teeth, but also is involved in blood clotting and nerve and muscle function.

Peptidase. An enzyme that splits simple peptides or their derivatives.

Peptide. Two or more amino acids combined in head-to-tail links. Generally larger than simple amino acids or the monoamines, the largest peptides discovered thus far have forty-four amino acids. Neuropeptides signal the body's endocrine glands to balance salt and water. Opiate peptides can help control pain and anxiety. The peptides work with amino acids. A peptide is present at two ten-thousandths of its partner amino acid or one hundredth of a monoamine.

Pituitary gland. The pea-sized gland situated at the base of the brain, once thought to be the master gland that gave "orders" to other glands. It is now known that the pituitary gland takes its orders from the hypothalamus (*see* Hypothalamus). The pituitary then sends out orders to the other glands in your body. The frontal lobe of the gland produces six hormones: growth hormone, which regulates growth; prolactin, which stimulates the breasts and has other functions as yet are not clearly understood; and four other hormones that stimulate the thyroid, adrenals, ovaries in women, and testes in men. The back lobe of the pituitary produces two hormones: antidiurectic hormone, which acts on the kidneys and regulates urine output, and oxytocin, which stimulates the contractions of the womb during childbirth.

Receptor. A protein molecule, which may also be composed of fat and carbohydrate, that resides on the surface or in the nucleus of a cell and recognizes and binds a specific molecule of appropriate size, shape, and charge.

Receptor binding assay. A technique to determine the presence and amount of a drug, neurotransmitter, or receptor in a biological system.

Releasing factors. Produced by the hypothalamus and then sent to the pituitary where they cause the release of appropriate hormones. Among those that have been found are luteinizing hormone-releasing hormone (LHRH), which affects the release of the sex hormones, and thyroid hormone–releasing factor (TRF), which affects the release of the thyroid hormone. Both LHRH and TRF have behavioral effects. LHRH, for example, enhances mating behavior. TRF can cause stimulation.

Serotonin. A neurotransmitter thought to play a role in temperature regulation, mood, and sleep.

Stroke. (*See* Cerebral vascular accident).

Substance P. A neurotransmitter believed to carry pain messages from the body to the brain and vice versa.

Sympathetic nervous system. Consists of nerve fibers that leave the brain and spinal cord, pass through the nerve cells clusters (ganglia), and are distributed to the heart, lungs, intestine, blood vessels, and sweat glands. In general, sympathetic nerves dilate the pupils, constrict small blood vessels, and increase heart rate. The system also involves circulating substances produced by the adrenal glands.

Synapse. The minute space between two neurons or between a neuron and an organ across which nerve impulses are chemically transmitted.

Thyroid gland. A butterfly-shaped gland located in the neck with a "wing" on either side of the windpipe. The gland produces thyroxine, which controls the rates of chemical reactions in the body. Generally, the more thyroxine, the faster the body works. Thyroxine needs iodine to function.

Vagus nerve. Literally the "wandering nerve" because it has such a wide distribution in the body, the vagus nerve connects the stomach to the brain and is involved in other autonomic functions such as breathing and heart rate.

Vasoactive intestinal peptide (VIP). A neurotransmitter present in both the gut and the brain. Its peripheral effects include lowering blood pressure by causing vasodilation, suppressing the secretion of stomach acid, and stimulating secretion in the small intestine and colon. VIP stimulates the release of a number of pituitary hormones, including growth hormone and prolactin, and may thus help to regulate the hormone glands. It also may play a part in arousal.

Index